JUN **1 4** 2019

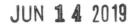

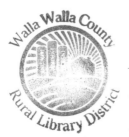

37 Jade Street

Walla Walla, WA 99362

KETO
DIET

ALSO BY DR. JOSH AXE

Eat Dirt

KETO
DIET

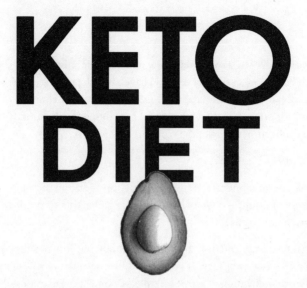

Your 30-Day Plan to Lose Weight,
Balance Hormones, Boost Brain Health,
and Reverse Disease

DR. JOSH AXE

Little, Brown Spark
New York Boston London

Little, Brown Spark
Hachette Book Group
1290 Avenue of the Americas, New York, NY 10104
littlebrownspark.com

First Edition: February 2019

Little, Brown Spark is an imprint of Little, Brown and Company, a division of Hachette Book Group, Inc. The Little, Brown Spark name and logo are trademarks of Hachette Book Group, Inc.

The publisher is not responsible for websites (or their content) that are not owned by the publisher.

The Hachette Speakers Bureau provides a wide range of authors for speaking events. To find out more, go to hachettespeakersbureau.com or call (866) 376-6591.

ISBN 978-0-316-52958-7
LCCN 2018957422

10 9 8 7 6 5 4 3 2 1

LSC-C

Printed in the United States of America

*This book is dedicated to my best friend, my wife, and the love of
my life, Chelsea Axe, and to my father God, for giving
me the platform and favor to create this book.*

Contents

PART IV

KETO DIET EATING

KETO
DIET

Finding a Better Way

Foolish the doctor who despises the knowledge acquired by the ancients.

— Hippocrates

*T*here *must be a better way*. I first had that thought as a thirteen-year-old kid in Troy, Ohio, when I discovered clumps of my mom's sandy-blond hair on our bathroom floor—a side effect of the chemotherapy that was poisoning her body in order to treat a cluster of cancer cells in her left breast and lymph nodes. The same unsettling thought struck again when my vibrant, athletic mom (a swim instructor and my school gym teacher) emerged from treatment seemingly cured of cancer but robbed of her spark, her energy, and her health.

There must be a better way.

At that age, I knew absolutely nothing about nutrition, but one public service message found its way into my adolescent brain: Soda is unhealthy. So I decided I would no longer drink it. This was the first time it occurred to me that food and diet might somehow be part of a "better way." If soda was bad for you, might other foods be, too—and might some be *good* for you as well?

For the next decade, my mom struggled with a range of health problems that left her feeling sick and tired all the time. Depression. Hypothyroidism. Constipation. Chronic fatigue syndrome. All this from a woman who, prior to treatment, could easily work a full-time job, care for her family, and then go for a workout or run and still feel energized. As I watched her health decline, an idea began to take hold, and over the years it continued to grow. I would become a doctor. I'd learn for myself why my mom had to sacrifice her health to treat her illness. And I'd try to find a better way.

By the time I was in my twenties, that dream was becoming a reality. I was attending chiropractic college in Florida, where I learned the foundations of nutrition. I also began training as a doctor of functional medicine and learning about ancient remedies. The wisdom of traditional Chinese medicine and Ayurvedic medicine made sense to me. These millennia-old practices worked with your body rather than against it. Instead of looking at an illness in isolation, the treatments took the whole person into consideration and aimed to heal the root cause of disease. They saw the forest *and* the trees, restoring overall health while eradicating illness. And they used food as medicine to bolster the body and create the optimal conditions for healing.

Nutrition was a key piece of the "better way" puzzle that was slowly coming together in my mind. As I read everything I could get my hands on about food and healing, I came across the ketogenic diet. I was blown away by the research. Here's a diet that actually transforms the way the body uses macronutrients, shifting your main fuel source from carbohydrates to fat. No other approach, short of fasting, can accomplish that. As a result, it can be a game changer for people who have struggled for years to lose weight, because it literally turns your body into a fat-burning machine. At the same time, the overall health implications are profound. It can reduce inflammation, balance vital hormones like insulin, and boost your brain health. During my research, I learned that the diet had already been used for decades to treat epilepsy and diabetes—and was being explored for other diseases as well, including cancer.

I was in that mode of research and discovery when I received a tearful call from my mom. "My oncologist told me they found a tumor on my lungs," she said, voice quavering. My stomach dropped. *No*, I thought, *not again*. My mom was my inspiration—and she'd already been through so much. I told her I loved her and would be there soon. The next day, I was on a plane to Ohio.

Back in my family home, my mom explained that her doctors had recommended surgery and radiation. I told her I believed there was a better way—one that would strengthen her body's innate healing mechanisms, support her overall health, and offer a sane, sustainable, scientifically sound approach to lifelong wellness.

Then I dove headlong into my research. I spent hundreds of hours reading about cancer and nutrition and herbs and antioxidants, and I reached out to some of the world's leading integrative medicine physicians for advice on nutrition and lifestyle changes that could support immunity and healing. Based on what I learned, we completely revamped my mom's diet.

We got rid of all the processed foods in her cupboards and filled her fridge with veggies, herbs, healthy protein, wholesome fat, and bone broth. I showed her how to make delicious vegetable juices with celery, spinach, cilantro, ginger, lemon, and beets. We bought wild salmon and cod liver oil, both of which are packed with inflammation-lowering omega-3 fatty acids. My mom began eating a variety of mushrooms, like shiitake and cordyceps and reishi, known as the mushroom of immortality in traditional Chinese medicine. She used herbs like milk thistle, known to detoxify the body, and turmeric, a potent anti-inflammatory that may play a role in reversing a variety of diseases, including cancer. We all but eliminated processed carbs and added sugar from her diet.

She made other healthy changes, too. She began getting lymphatic massage and chiropractic care; praying and doing positive, healing affirmations; and using essential oils like frankincense, which relieves stress and anxiety, supports immunity, and contains antitumor properties. She'd been diagnosed with cancer, but you'd never know it. As the weeks rolled by, she began feeling more energetic than she had in years, her depression lifted, and she lost twenty-two pounds.

When she went to her doctor four months later for a CT scan, he could hardly believe the images. Her tumor had shrunk to half its original size—without any chemo or radiation. Nine months after her diagnosis, she was in almost complete remission. Now, thirteen years later, she's cancer-free. She water-skis, runs 5K races, and keeps up with her grandkids. She says she feels better now, in her sixties, than she did in her thirties.

I'm not suggesting that those who've been diagnosed with cancer ignore their doctors' advice. Life-altering decisions should be made only with the help of trusted health-care practitioners and based on the unique characteristics of each individual diagnosis. But bolstering your body's defenses with nutrition makes sense no matter what health challenge you're facing. The diet that helped my mom beat cancer was a modified version of the keto protocol I lay out in this book. For me, the experience was pivotal. I had all the proof I needed. I had discovered a better way.

ANCIENT NUTRITION IN A MODERN WORLD

My keto diet program isn't a gimmicky fad, nor is its sole purpose to help you slim down. It's a scientific way to lower inflammation, correct hormonal imbalances, jump-start your weight loss, and transform your health, giving you the best shot at a disease-free future. It doesn't involve hunger or deprivation or calorie counting. It's a high-fat, moderate-protein, very-low-carb approach—a unique mix that accomplishes something no other diet can: It fundamentally changes the way your body burns calories. By shifting the source of energy your brain and muscles utilize from carbs to fat, it forces your body to let go of that stubborn spare tire around your belly—the fat that's frustrating from a cosmetic standpoint and largely responsible for the health problems that go hand in hand with being overweight. As a result, my keto diet program is the one diet that can work for you when every other diet has failed.

The approach is grounded in science, but it's based on the way humans have been eating since the beginning of time. Our ancestors didn't have access to grocery store shelves overflowing with cereal, chips, and macaroni and cheese, nor was food available 24/7. Their sustenance came straight from nature—from the organic plants, herbs, berries, nuts, and free-range meat in their surroundings—so its availability was up to nature's whims, and they experienced cycles of feast and famine. Alternating between plentiful periods when food was abundant and challenging phases when it was scarce had an upside. During the intermittent famines, their bodies went into *ketosis*, the health-promoting state in which you burn fat, rather than carbohydrates, for fuel.

You can get into ketosis with fasting. Or you can get there with the ketogenic diet. The approach was discovered in the 1920s. Doctors working at Johns Hopkins University and the Mayo Clinic were treating patients with disparate problems—intractable seizure disorders and diabetes. They had learned that fasting helped alleviate their patients' symptoms, but the symptoms returned once the patients started eating again. So, independently, the researchers at each institution began manipulating their patients' diets to try to mimic a fasting state. When they cut carbs to almost zero, their patients went into ketosis. The seizures stopped and their blood sugar normalized. The ketogenic diet was born.

My keto diet program is based on the well-established science behind that breakthrough discovery. Its macronutrient combination triggers the same healthy metabolic condition as fasting. So while you're eating satisfying, nutritious meals, you reap the health benefits of abstinence: You burn fat for fuel, normalize hormone levels, slash inflammation, and give your body the opportunity to heal.

Let me say this again: My keto diet plan doesn't entail deprivation, much less starvation. The plan is built around delicious foods that melt off fat, reduce your sugar cravings, and help you feel mentally sharp, energetic, and sated. Like fasting, it's not meant to be a long-term approach. But in this day and age, when everything from stress to environmental toxins can throw your system out of whack, my keto diet program is a scientifically proven way to reboot your body by resetting and stabilizing its basic biochemical functions. Even better: There's a way to benefit from ketosis for the long term, an approach known as keto cycling that I explain in detail in the upcoming pages.

THE BIG, FAT TRUTH

You undoubtedly already know that the United States is the most overweight industrialized nation in the world. No one wants to be overweight—and people who are have tried diet after diet to get their weight under control. Despite those sincere attempts, we're heavier than ever. In 1960, 31 percent of U.S. adults were overweight and 13 percent were obese. Today, a whopping 70 percent are overweight—

and more than a third fall into the obese category, where the risks of weight-related health problems are the most dire.

Gaining a pound or two a year has become the norm—an accepted and expected side effect of aging. But here's the thing: Age-related weight gain *isn't* inevitable. It's actually a sign of imbalance, in both your external lifestyle (too much food, too little physical activity) and your internal physical environment—specifically, hormones that have gone haywire. Those accruing pounds so many people take for granted are truly dangerous, putting you at increased risk of serious health problems that limit your ability to feel and function your best—from high blood pressure, heart disease, and diabetes to sleep apnea, arthritis, and hormonal issues, like polycystic ovary syndrome, which can make it difficult to get pregnant. Excess weight also boosts your odds of developing certain types of cancer, including breast, colon, and gallbladder.

There are a number of causes for the obesity epidemic, but the processed carbs that form the basis of most Americans' diets are largely to blame. Heavily processed foods contain "obesogens"—toxic chemicals that make us fat—and hidden sugars that hook our brains, mess with our blood sugar, energy, and mood, and leave us craving more. After watching thousands of patients—including my wife, Chelsea, who lost those last stubborn ten pounds, balanced her hormones, and got lean on the ketogenic diet—and experiencing the program for myself (it made me leaner than ever), I can say with certainty that the fastest way to lose weight and keep it off for good is by radically slashing carbs, at least temporarily, so you start incinerating your body's deep, unreachable fat stores. The ketogenic diet is the only approach that's specifically designed to achieve that goal.

The secret to my keto diet program's effectiveness is an optimal mix of macronutrients: high amounts of healthy fat, moderate protein, and low, low carbs. The idea of eating fat to shed weight might sound counterintuitive. But the right kinds of fat, studies show, actually help you lose stubborn body fat. My keto diet plan is built around healthy fats—the type in avocados, coconut oil, olive oil, and salmon. Those fats are actually good for your brain and heart. They taste good, too.

The keto diet program is lower in carbs than most low-carb eating plans. It's super low carb—about 30 grams a day. Without the grains and starchy vegetables and fruit that the body typically relies on for fuel, your body starts utilizing fat within three or four days. You enter ketosis and begin torching the stubborn pudge that's collected around your belly or thighs or back.

That metabolic state is also deeply restorative and triggers a cascade of healthy changes:

- Your body releases less insulin, so two things happen: You store less fat and your blood sugar levels normalize—slashing your risk of diabetes.
- Levels of triglycerides and bad (LDL) cholesterol fall, while good (HDL) cholesterol rises—all factors that protect the health of your heart.
- Your natural ability to fight cancer improves, because sugar is the fuel cancer cells need to survive. Studies indicate that the very-low-carb ketogenic diet may actually starve and shrink tumors.
- You achieve optimal brain function by improving the ability of mitochondria—tiny organs in cells that transform fuel into energy—to do their job. In fact, promising new research shows that by maintaining healthy functioning in the brain's energy centers, ketosis may protect against an array of devastating neurological disorders, from Alzheimer's, Parkinson's, and epilepsy to headaches, traumatic brain injuries, and sleep disorders.

READY, SET, KETO

There are a number of approaches to the ketogenic diet, but mine is unique. It's designed not just to put your body into fat-burning ketosis but also to create the optimal environment for healing. As a result, my keto program isn't all about bacon and butter. It's about giving your body the veggies, herbs, vitamins, and minerals that are the basic building blocks of health and healing.

The upcoming chapters contain all the information you need to fully understand my keto diet and get the most out of the next thirty days—and the rest of your life. Part I forms the foundation. I explain in an easy-to-digest way how the keto diet works and why it is so effective. I cover the biggest keto diet mistakes I see other people make, helping you avoid common pitfalls that can undermine the diet's effectiveness. I share powerful stories of people, including my wife and my patients, who've gone through my Keto360 program, which features the keto diet plan in this book as well as online support. (For more information on my in-depth Keto360 program, visit www.draxe.com/keto-diet-keto360.) Plus, I fill you in on the top keto diet foods, supplements, exercises, and essential oils—and I include a detailed shopping list and even cover how to eat out and travel while going keto.

In Part II, we dig deeper. I explain how the keto diet program transforms the health of your whole body down to your cells and mitochondria by reducing inflammation, producing ketones, and balancing insulin. I'll cover how you can boost the health of your brain, hormones, and metabolism and fight cancer with a ketogenic diet.

Part III gives you five different short-term keto plans to choose from based on your health goals and how deep and far you want to go with keto: a beginners' plan, an advanced plan that includes intermittent fasting, a plan for vegans, a plan for those looking to boost their collagen and fight aging, and a keto cancer plan. And I make it all super easy by giving you access to more than eighty delicious keto recipes.

Regardless of which plan you choose, you'll need a way to incorporate the keto diet into your life for the long term. That's where the final program in Part III comes in. The Forever Keto Cycling Plan is a sustainable approach that allows you to go in and out of ketosis over and over, keeping your body trim, youthful, and healthy for years to come.

I'm excited you're here—and grateful you've made the choice to join my mission to create a more robust and healthy world. If you want to support your brain and neurological health, balance your hormones, improve your digestive health, lose weight, burn fat, bolster your energy, and feel your best, my keto diet program is for you. It's time to put the frustration and disappointment of failed diets and deteriorating health behind us. Welcome to a better way.

PART I

Meet the Keto Diet

CHAPTER 1

The Diet That Works When Nothing Else Will

The Need for Ancient Nutrition in Today's Toxic World

In my twenty years of helping patients, friends, and family improve their health, one of the facts about diet that surprises them most is that fat is critical to the human body and carbohydrates play a minor role. We've been duped into believing that carbs are good and fat is bad. I'm here to tell you: That's not true. Of the three macronutrients that food contains—fat, protein, and carbohydrates—carbs are the only one known by scientists and doctors to be nonessential.

For proof you need look no further than your own body. If we exclude water, the average human body is made up of 73 percent fat, 25 percent protein, and 2 percent carbs. See that ratio? Mostly fat. Almost no carbs. Fat is crucial for the optimal functioning of the 37 trillion cells in your body. It protects your organs, supplies energy to your body and brain, and plays a vital role in hormone signaling, including insulin, estrogen, and testosterone. Not only that, but approximately 60 percent of your brain and nervous system is made up of fat,[1] and 25 percent of that is cholesterol. And at just three pounds, a fraction of your overall weight, your brain utilizes 20 percent of your body's metabolic energy and oxygen.

In this book, I'm going to show you how consuming more fat and fewer carbs—the opposite of what you've always been told—is the dietary strategy that can transform your health. In my functional medicine clinic, I've seen proof that the unique high-fat, very-low-carb approach I describe in *Keto Diet* can change people's lives.

One patient's doctor prescribed a no-fat diet for heart disease. By the time he came to me, his hair was thinning, his muscles were wasting, and his liver was failing. I put him on a high-fat ketogenic diet and his hair grew back, his muscle mass rebounded, and his cardiovascular system became so healthy he was able to go off all his heart medications.

Another patient had been struggling with infertility for years, the result of hormones that were badly out of whack. She had hypothyroidism and polycystic ovary syndrome. I prescribed a strict thirty-day keto diet, followed by a less regimented keto cycling plan. Two months later, her hormones were healthy—and she was pregnant.

I consulted with an MD friend who was diagnosed with cancer of the spine. His doctors had told him his only hope was chemo, and even then, his prognosis was grim. I suggested he try a strict ketogenic diet. That was eight years ago. He's been cancer-free ever since.

My keto diet program has worked for hundreds of my patients, and it can work for you, too. But first you need to forget most of the conventional rules you've been taught about what you're supposed to eat, because most of those rules are dead wrong.

You've been told that the key to weight loss is eating less and exercising more.

It's not.

You've been told that eating fat will make you fat and contribute to heart disease.

It won't.

You've been told that your lack of results is due to your lack of willpower.

It isn't.

You've been told that your hormone imbalance, digestive issues, pain, or other medical conditions are incurable, and no diet can fix them.

Not true.

We now know that the composition of your diet — the mix of *high-quality* fat, protein, and carbohydrates — rather than how carefully you count calories or how much you burn off with exercise is the key to losing weight and improving your health. A 100-calorie snack pack of cookies has a dramatically different effect on your body than half an avocado or a small handful of almonds with about the same number of calories. *Keto Diet* is based on that radical shift in understanding about what makes diets succeed or fail — as well as on my longtime experience as a doctor of functional medicine and clinical nutritionist, treating hundreds of patients who have tried to follow the conventional rules and wound up heavier, sicker, and more tired than before.

Not all ketogenic diets are created equal. To get the most out of this new approach to looking and feeling your best, the specific foods you eat are vitally important. *Keto Diet* explains my unique, über-healthy, super-clean take on the concept, which will help you avoid common pitfalls of other ketogenic diets, get the most nutrition out of every bite, and optimize the benefits of this game-changing plan. Over the years, I've discovered the ideal mix of key nutrients, along with the best, most wholesome sources of those nutrients. My patients who follow this approach are able to reduce inflammation, balance their hormones, and lose the stubborn body fat that has been making them unhappy and unwell. After years of trying, they finally attain their health and wellness goals.

DR. AXE KETO VS. STANDARD KETO

Dr. Axe Keto	Standard Keto
Loads of veggies	Few veggies
Organic meat	Conventional meat
High in collagen	No collagen
Nutrient-dense foods	Focus on butter/bacon
Alkalizing	Acidic
Anti-inflammatory herbs and spices	No herbs/spices

If you're like most of my patients, you can expect to lose an average of fifteen to eighteen pounds in your thirty days on my keto diet plan—and you'll continue losing afterward if you stick with the Forever Keto Cycling program, which is designed to achieve and maintain optimal health and weight for the long term. You won't be eating the same boring old foods, by the way. You'll love the simple recipes for dishes like Keto Pancakes, Keto Florentine Pizza, and Keto Fudge. Did you ever think you could lose weight by eating food like that?

What you can expect to *gain* on my keto diet program is equally life changing: increased energy, vitality, and mental clarity. Those of you who have struggled with conditions like diabetes, polycystic ovary syndrome, epilepsy, infertility, heart disease, thyroid disease, digestive problems, multiple sclerosis, migraine headaches, and autoimmune disease will likely see a dramatic improvement. And even though it's controversial to say that dietary changes can improve Alzheimer's, autism, and cancer, I'm here to tell you that I've seen significant healing with the *right type* of keto diet. Even if you've become so dispirited by failed attempts to heal a chronic disorder or lose weight that you've given up trying, there's hope in these pages. This keto diet plan can work when nothing else can.

KETO MYTHS

KETO IS A HIGH-FAT, HIGH-PROTEIN DIET.
KETO IS FOR WEIGHT LOSS ONLY.
YOU CAN'T EXERCISE ON KETO.
YOU WILL LOSE MUSCLE MASS.
YOU WILL ALWAYS HAVE LOW ENERGY.
KETO IS THE SAME FOR MEN AND WOMEN.
YOU HAVE TO FAST INTERMITTENTLY.
YOU CAN'T DRINK ALCOHOL.

NEW SCIENCE SUPPORTS A RETURN TO ANCIENT NUTRITION

My keto diet program isn't magic. Its effectiveness is based on sound, well-known scientific principles of physiology. With every other weight-loss plan, including low-carb approaches, you burn carbohydrates, or glucose — the sugar that's created when you metabolize carbs — for fuel, just like you would if you were eating a regular American diet. But my keto diet program's unique mix of high fat, moderate protein, and extremely low carbs triggers a vital biochemical shift in your metabolism. Instead of burning glucose for fuel, within four days you begin burning fat. Think about that. After just a few days, you start incinerating the stubborn love handles and belly fat you may have tried to get rid of for years. You actually continue burning fat while you sleep, so you wake up in the morning looking and feeling slimmer and leaner. No other diet, except fasting, does that. The keto diet is in a category by itself.

Compared to the way most people eat today, this approach to peak health is revolutionary — and yet it's a return to the time-tested nutritional principles of our ancestors. The basic biology of the ketogenic diet comes from the days when our ancestors hunted and gathered their food. They didn't eat three meals a day. They didn't have grocery stores stocked with every imaginable form of nourishment or pantries filled with packaged snacks to grab the moment they felt a twinge of hunger. Instead, their survival depended on what they could forage or hunt. Even after they began to learn how to grow their own food, they ate sporadically. They might have had a large midmorning breakfast, then skipped a meal or two — or even gone several days eating hardly anything at all. Our ancestors' relationship with food was simple and straightforward. They ate what they had on hand. When food was scarce they went hungry. But intermittent hunger, it turns out, was surprisingly good for them.

You've probably heard that fasting can be beneficial for your health — but you might not know why. It's actually quite simple: The human body can store only about twenty-four hours' worth of glucose, the quickest, most accessible form of fuel. Unless you consume carbo-hydrates, your body is incapable of making more. When your natural supply of glucose is depleted, your cells turn to the next best thing and begin burning fat for fuel. Your system goes into a deeply restorative state known as *ketosis*.

5 STEPS TO KETOSIS-FUELED WEIGHT LOSS

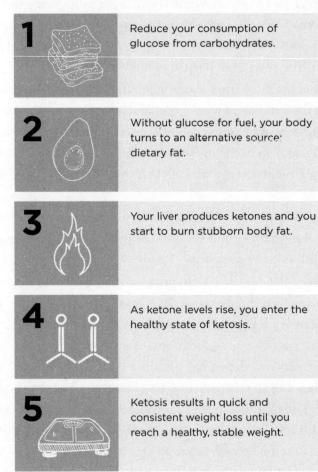

1 Reduce your consumption of glucose from carbohydrates.

2 Without glucose for fuel, your body turns to an alternative source: dietary fat.

3 Your liver produces ketones and you start to burn stubborn body fat.

4 As ketone levels rise, you enter the healthy state of ketosis.

5 Ketosis results in quick and consistent weight loss until you reach a healthy, stable weight.

During ketosis, all sorts of good things start to happen. As you uti-lize fatty acids for energy, the deep wells of stubborn fat around your body start to disappear—making you leaner and healthier, since body fat plays a role in heart disease, diabetes, insulin resistance, and other metabolic disorders. Your brain benefits, too—and the effects are tangible: improved memory and mental clarity and less frequent headaches. While ketosis torches fat, it also brings insulin into balance—and taming out-of-control insulin has a domino-like effect on dozens of other dangerous conditions, like diabetes, hormone-related issues from PMS to low testosterone, and chronic inflammation, the culprit that drives conditions like arthritis, irritable bowel syndrome, chronic pain, and Alzheimer's.

Back in the era when humans didn't know where their next meal was coming from, our ancestors' bodies functioned like hybrid cars, using carbs for fuel when they had food on hand, then shifting to fat during times of famine. The pattern of cycling in and out of ketosis throughout their lives kept them, based on skeletal evidence, lean and free of the diseases that plague our modern society. And it can work for you, too.

Keto Diet's thirty-day plan is designed to jump-start your weight loss and reset your health by keeping you in a steady state of ketosis. Afterward, the Forever Keto Cycling Plan allows you to naturally move in and out of ketosis, just like the ancients, for the rest of your life. As a result, the keto diet program is the single most reliable way to lose weight fast and forever, get out of the yo-yo dieting rut, and change your health for good.

WHY OTHER DIETS DON'T WORK AND THIS ONE DOES

Despite the fact that doctors and public health officials have been waging a war on obesity since the 1980s, and Americans spend $66 billion every year trying to be loyal foot soldiers and shed their excess pounds, we're fighting a losing battle. As a country, we've become steadily fatter and less healthy. In 1980, fewer than half of adults in the United States were overweight or obese. Now, more than 70 percent fit that description—and nearly 8 percent of them fall into a category known as "extreme obesity," with a body mass index (BMI) of 40 or more.

It's a worrisome, even heartbreaking trend. Carrying extra weight is linked to all sorts of negative health outcomes. And there are signs it may be getting worse. According to recent research, the number of active dieters has declined by 10 percent since 2015. Why would overweight people abandon their efforts to try to get healthy? Some health experts theorize that fewer people are dieting because the size-acceptance movement is reducing the stigma of being overweight. But I believe it has to do with our flawed approach to dieting itself. After repeated attempts to lose weight, more and more people have simply reached the point of diet fatigue. And who could blame them? If you try and fail over and over, at some point you're going to fail to try again.

Fortunately, we now understand the reasons that the majority of people on traditional diets regain their lost weight within one to five years. It's important for you to understand why your past attempts at getting healthy and losing weight have failed, too — and why my keto diet program can help you succeed:

You start burning fewer calories because your body thinks it's starving. Recent research has shown that when you lose 10 percent of your body weight on a conventional diet, your metabolism slows.[2] In fact, the number of calories you burn during the day can drop by 30 to 40 percent—an amount that's enough to completely undermine your efforts to maintain your new weight. And your metabolism may not rebound for years. In order to keep the weight off, you have to eat even less, a long-term challenge that, for most people, is unachievable.

How the keto diet is different: By changing the macronutrient composition of your diet, you prevent your metabolism from taking a hit. A 2012 study published in the *Journal of the American Medical Association*[3] had participants lose 10 to 15 percent of their body weight before going on one of three different maintenance diets—low fat, with about 60 percent of daily calories from carbs; low glycemic index, with about 40 percent from healthy carbs like whole grains and vegetables; and very low carb, with just 10 percent of daily calories from carbs—a carbohydrate level similar to that of my keto diet program. After each diet period, the researchers tested people's metabolic rates and found that the very-low-carb diet prevented the metabolic slowdown often seen after weight loss. In fact, people on the very-low-carb plan burned an average of 325 calories a day *more* than those on the low-fat diet—about the amount you'd burn during a decent workout—and about 150 calories more than those on the low-glycemic-index diet. In other words, unlike every other diet out there, the keto diet keeps your metabolism humming at a healthy rate so you can continue to eat a normal amount without gaining weight.

You get way too hungry. Nearly every weight-loss program throughout history—from the grapefruit diet to the vinegar diet to the cigarette diet (yes, that was once a trend), right on up to most of the popular approaches today—is based on the flawed math that experts have always thought was irrefutable: Eat less + burn more = weight loss. True, that equation does help you shed pounds. *At first.* Then something that no one could have predicted begins happening. When you lose weight, your body kicks into starvation mode and launches potent countermeasures designed to prevent additional weight loss. The more weight you lose, the more fiercely your body fights back. And its tactics are brutal. Not only does your metabolism slow, but your primal self-preservation system starts churning out a number of powerful hunger- and satiety-related hormones. Ghrelin, the hunger hormone, shoots up, increasing your desire to eat and triggering cravings for high-calorie, carb-laden goodies. And leptin, the hormone that helps you feel full, doesn't kick in as quickly—so you feel less satisfied with a reasonable amount of food. As your satiety off switch dims and your appetite spikes, every day becomes a battle; your body is unconsciously pushing you to eat, while you're desperately trying to resist. That's why as many as 95 percent of people who lose weight on conventional diets regain it all—and often more—within five years. If you're fighting against your body, it's a battle you can't win.

How the keto diet is different: One remarkable aspect of my keto plan is how incredibly satisfying it is. Patients are always struck by how full they feel. One meal keeps them satisfied for three or four hours. Increasing your fat intake fends off that gnawing feeling of most diets, because fat takes a long time to digest; it releases energy slowly over time, so your energy doesn't spike, then plummet, as it does when you burn glucose. And burning fat for fuel instead of carbs seems to short-circuit the body's starvation-mode mechanism. Australian researchers reported in 2013 that even when study subjects lost 13 percent of their initial weight—a significant amount—on a ketogenic diet, their levels of ghrelin, the hunger hormone, didn't rise as they typically do in people who lose weight.[4] When you shed pounds through ketosis, your body doesn't fight back.

Nonstop calorie counting is tedious and keeps you focused on deprivation. In 1990, the nation passed the Nutrition Labeling and Education Act—and as soon as people could see the number of calories in foods, they began counting them and cutting them. Diets became about restriction, denial, and deprivation—powerful emotional triggers for cravings. Not surprisingly, this punishing approach isn't sustainable. And calorie counting has another fatal flaw. It encourages you to avoid satisfying sources of healthy fat, because fat has more calories than carbs—9 versus 4 per gram. Many people who are overly focused on calories make the mistake of turning to high-carb, low-calorie processed foods in place of satisfying fat—and here's what happens: Processed carbs digest quickly into sugar and cause your body to release more insulin, the hormone produced by the pancreas that regulates the amount of glucose in your blood. And insulin prompts your body to store calories as fat. So the more low-calorie carbs you consume, the more fat you pack on.

How the keto diet is different: It's not about calories at all. When you're eating superhealthy sources of fat and very few carbs, your meals are satisfying, so you naturally eat an appropriate number of calories and lose weight without trying. Just as important, fat doesn't raise insulin. We've all been told that a calorie is a calorie is a calorie, but that's not true. A sweet granola bar and a small handful of nuts have about the same number of calories, but a sugar-laden bar causes a dramatic insulin surge while nuts cause none. By eating more fat, you actually burn more fat and store less fat. How cool is that?

You eat the wrong foods. A number of packaged foods—and even some fruits and vegetables—contain obesogens, or chemicals that encourage fat storage. These sneaky substances mess with your hormones and can make it tough to lose weight and keep it off. Artificial sweeteners like aspartame and saccharine, monosodium glutamate (often found in Chinese food), and high-fructose corn syrup all fall into this fat-promoting category. And a chemical known as BPA (bisphenol-A), which is used in plastic packaging and canned foods, is an obesogen as well. But even healthy foods can be a problem. Conventionally grown fruits and vegetables contain pesticides and fungicides that can change the way your hormones function and promote obesity. If you don't try to avoid obesogens, you'll undermine your efforts to get healthy.

How the keto diet is different: My plan includes only clean, whole-some, chemical-free foods — organic vegetables grown without pesti-cides: organic, grass-fed meat; wild-caught fish; cage-free eggs; and organic, high-quality fats and oils. You won't eat anything that comes from a can or contains artificial sweeteners. My keto diet program is free of chemicals that can promote weight gain — and chock-full of nutrients that promote robust good health and support weight loss.

WHY THE KETO DIET IS A HEALTHY OPTION FOR EVERYONE

The ketogenic diet is the only eating plan that shifts your fuel source from carbs to fat — and it's hard to overestimate the beneficial effects of that single change. Utilizing fat for fuel makes you slimmer and healthier — and addresses a newly recognized health scourge that is rapidly becoming the "new obesity" epidemic. So-called overfat, a condition in which, although your weight is normal, your body is dis-proportionately made up of fat as opposed to lean muscle tissue and bone, affects roughly 80 percent of women and 90 percent of men in the United States.[5]

Even if you don't need to lose weight, there's a good chance you're carrying around too much body fat — a hidden hazard that can silently increase your risk of heart disease, stroke, cancer, diabetes, arthritis, gout, lung disease, and sleep apnea. A large-scale 2016 study published in the *Annals of Internal Medicine* found that people with a high body-fat percentage were at an increased risk of dying, regardless of their BMI.[6]

In other words, the number on the scale doesn't adequately reflect your general wellness, since it doesn't measure what's underneath your skin. The amount of fat inside your body, even if you can't see it, can make or break your health.

My keto diet's specific macronutrient profile is the only one that quickly and effectively addresses the new epidemic of overfat, along with all its inherent risks. And that's just one crucial aspect of the diet's extensive impact. Here's what makes my keto diet's very-low-carb, high-fat profile such a radical departure from anything else you've ever tried — and why it just might change your life.

Carbs make you fat and sick

Most people eat a diet that's made up of roughly 50 percent carbs, 34 percent fat, and 16 percent protein.[7] Because your body processes carbs much faster than protein or fat, your energy boomerangs up and down all day. And along with these energy spikes and dips, carbs flood your bloodstream with sugar, triggering two harmful responses. First, high blood sugar prompts your pancreas to release a flood of insulin — a hormone David Ludwig, MD, an endocrinologist and professor of nutrition at Harvard School of Public Health, calls "the ultimate fat-cell fertilizer," because it instructs your body to store calories as fat.[8] The result: Your fat cells increase in number and size.

As if that weren't bad enough, when insulin ushers calories into your fat cells, it closes the door, trapping those calories inside. With those precious sources of fuel locked inside your fat cells, there's too little glucose available to power your brain and muscles. Your brain, sensing a food shortage, stimulates the sensation of hunger. So, according to Dr. Ludwig and others, it's not overeating that makes us fat. Processed, sugary foods have programmed our fat cells to grow, and that makes us overeat. In other words, low-fat, highly processed sugary snacks and starches are actually one important cause of the obesity epidemic.

At the same time, the carb-induced sugar that's left floating around your bloodstream causes your body to launch an inflammatory immune reaction to get rid of the sugar—and inflammation, as I've mentioned, has been implicated in a number of serious health conditions, like Alzheimer's and cancer. Inflammation is your body's response to outside threats. When it's used to fight off an infection in a cut on your finger, it can be lifesaving. When it becomes chronic because of problems like high blood sugar or plaque in your arteries, it's like a four-alarm fire in your body, damaging tissues and wreaking havoc on organs.

Nutrient-dense fat keeps you healthy

The low-fat craze that began in the 1970s was based on flawed but well-meaning logic: Since a gram of fat has more than twice as many calories as a gram of protein or carbohydrates, eating less fat, experts theorized, should be an easy way to lose weight. Pretty soon, fat-free products were everywhere—and guess what they contained? Refined carbohydrates and added sugars, ingredients that prompt the release of insulin and thereby promote fat storage. As a result, the low-fat craze helped create the obesity epidemic.

Now the tide has started to turn. In the last decade, a number of studies have vindicated dietary fat. A groundbreaking paper published in the esteemed *New England Journal of Medicine* several years ago compared overweight people who ate a low-fat diet, a moderate-fat Mediterranean diet, or a high-fat diet.[9] The trial lasted two years—a remarkable amount of time in the realm of diet studies and long enough to make its findings highly reliable. The researchers discovered that people on the high-fat diet not only lost the most weight, they also had the most favorable changes in heart disease–related risk factors, like triglycerides and HDL—and the participants who had diabetes had better blood sugar control. Eating fat, the study showed, was actually very good for participants' health.

Surprised? Don't be. By now we know that healthy dietary fat has a multitude of benefits—and my approach to the keto diet includes only the most nutrient-rich fats available. For instance, my keto diet, like our ancient ancestors' diets, is free of hydrogenated oils, and here's why:

During processing, these oils undergo structural changes and become oxidized, and oxidized oils lead to inflammation in your body. All the healthy fats in my keto diet program come from the most nutritious sources, and many are packed with other superhealthy vitamins, minerals, and fat-soluble nutrients.

Just as it's good to eat a variety of veggies so you get an array of phytochemicals and nutrients, it's important to eat a range of types of healthy fat, because each type offers different benefits. We'll dive deeper into the specific benefits of fats in future chapters, but here's a quick overview:

- Saturated fats make up a significant proportion of our cells' membranes, so they're vital for the health of every cell in our bodies, particularly our brain cells. Good sources are grass-fed animal products.

- Medium-chain fatty acids are the easiest type of fat for your body to metabolize and burn as fuel. They come from sources like unrefined coconut oil and palm oil.

- Omega-3 and omega-6 fatty acids are important for keeping inflammation in your body in check. The nutritious sources of these fats are wild-caught fish, like salmon, as well as flaxseeds, chia seeds, and hempseeds and oils like cod liver and flax. Seaweeds, which have been used as medicine for centuries, contain anti-inflammatory omega-3 fatty acids as well—plus so much more. Seaweed is such a nutrition powerhouse I think of it as superseaweed.

- Omega-9 monounsaturated fats lubricate your body's joints and support hormone health. My keto diet program encourages lots of delicious omega-9-rich foods, like avocados, nuts, seeds, and olives.

- Cholesterol from pasture-raised organic egg yolks can actually, despite what you've been told in the past, improve your good HDL cholesterol, hormonal health, and brain neurotransmitters.

If you want to jump-start your journey to lifelong good health, my high-fat, very-low-carb keto diet is the place to begin. By putting your body into a state of ketosis, the program offers widespread healing. It gives your pancreas, the organ that processes carbs, a chance to rest and

TOP 12 HIGH-FAT KETO FOODS

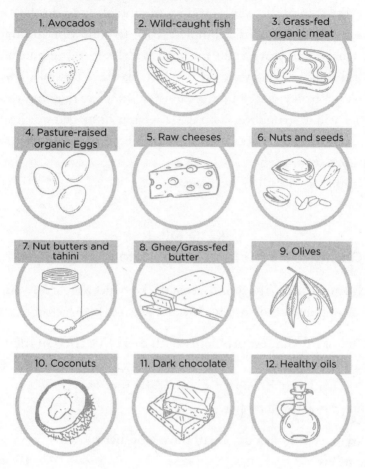

rejuvenate. It allows your body to break down scar tissue and helps your system identify and get rid of unhealthy cells that have accrued DNA damage and could lead to cancer. Ketosis is the most effective way to begin full-body healing.

Now that you understand the basics of my keto diet program, in the upcoming pages I'll walk you step by step through the whys and hows of the approach. In my functional medicine practice, I treat my patients as I would my own family members. I give them recipes and shopping lists—just as I did with my mom when she was fighting cancer and all the health issues that cropped up after she was treated the first time. I point out the common pitfalls of the ketogenic approach and help them problem solve their unique challenges. I let them know that I'm with them every step of the way—and it's my intention to do the same in this book. Just as I created a complete, easy-to-follow program for my mom, I have one that's right for you, with everything you need to make it fit into your lifestyle with as little hassle as possible. The keto diet isn't a journey you're taking alone. It's one we're going to share. Whether you're struggling with extra weight or diabetes or just don't feel your absolute best, I believe my keto diet program has the potential to transform your life.

It's time for a health breakthrough.

KETO QUIZ:
Could You Benefit from My Keto Diet Program?

Take this quick true/false quiz to see if the keto diet is right for you. After each true response, read on to understand why my keto diet plan can help.

1. **One of my biggest problems with diets I've tried in the past is hunger.**   T   F

   Thanks to its high-fat, low-carb profile, you won't get hungry on my keto diet.

2. **No matter what I do, I still have a belly or love handles.**   T   F

   The very-low-carb keto diet puts your body into ketosis and you start burning fat for fuel. Within days, you'll see that stubborn fat start to disappear.

3. **I notice my energy can be up and down during the day, and I may have a blood sugar imbalance.**   T   F

   Carbs are responsible for the spikes and dips of energy. When you reduce carbs and eat plenty of healthy fat, you can lower your blood sugar and bring insulin into balance.

4. **I often feel sluggish and mentally foggy.**   T   F

   Blame carbs. The ups and downs of blood sugar leave most

people feeling lethargic. The high-fat keto diet is great for your brain, which loves to use fat as fuel.

5. **Cancer runs in my family and I want to do everything I can to protect myself.**   **T   F**

    There are promising studies showing that the state of ketosis might rid the body of damaged cells that can lead to cancer.

6. **I'm struggling with hormonal issues (a thyroid condition, polycystic ovary syndrome, premenstrual syndrome, menopausal symptoms, low testosterone).**   **T   F**

    When insulin is rampant in your system, it also affects every other hormone in your body. By reducing your carb intake, you reduce insulin, which can help you get hormonal problems under control.

7. **My memory isn't as good as it used to be and I don't feel like my brain is performing at a high level.**   **T   F**

    Studies show that the ketogenic diet supports optimal brain functioning and can improve memory.

8. **I have digestive issues and/or yeast and candida growth.**   **T   F**

    The very low sugar content of the keto diet helps reverse gut issues and candida growth. At the same time, my keto diet plan contains tons of nonstarchy produce, which means it also gives your body prebiotics in the form of fiber. Prebiotics feed probiotics, the substances that keep your gut healthy.

9. **I have frequent pain in my joints and/or low back or neck.**   **T   F**

    Because the keto diet reduces inflammation, it also can reduce achiness all over your body.

10. **I have trouble sleeping or getting quality sleep.   T   F**

    Overeating carbs in the evening can be a cause of insomnia, as can insulin surges.

11. **I have food sensitivities and a weak immune system.** **T   F**

    Some of the most common food sensitivities come from so-called healthy carbs, like wheat, barley, and rye. The keto diet eliminates many sources of food sensitivities. At the same time, some food sensitivities are driven by the bacteria in your gut. By improving the health of your gut bacteria, the keto diet offers protection from food sensitivities as well.

12. **I have neurological issues and/or migraine headaches.** **T   F**

    The ketogenic diet was originally created to treat epilepsy, one type of neurological problem. It's been shown to help with headaches and is good for a wide range of neurological issues, from Parkinson's to Alzheimer's.

CHAPTER 2

The Keto Diet Advantage

The Remarkable Ways Ketosis Can Transform Your Health

Now that you know a little about how my keto diet program works, I'm going to share what it does for your health. This is where things get exciting. When you hear the word "diet" you probably think "weight loss." Period. But medical studies are proving that the ketogenic diet can not only help you lose weight remarkably fast but also boost your brain health, balance gut bacteria, reduce inflammation, fight cancer, balance hormones, and do a whole lot more. When I say it's the diet that can work when nothing else will, I mean it. Dozens of studies have revealed just how powerful this approach is for transforming your health.

The ketogenic diet is in a league of its own because it essentially hacks your body in a way no other diet can: It puts you into ketosis — so you stop burning sugar for energy and start burning fat. Here's the analogy I often use with patients: Say you want to build a campfire that will burn slowly, throw off consistent heat, and last a long time. You have three choices for fuel: kindling, logs, or coal. Kindling catches fire quickly and burns out fast. Logs burn longer, once they're finally lit. But the fuel that will give you the longest, steadiest, most satisfying burn is coal. The problem is, it's harder to get coal to light.

It's the same in your body. There are three types of fuel you can use for energy. Carbs are like kindling. They "catch fire" quickly and give you instant energy, but they burn off fast—so your energy crashes a couple of hours after you eat them, triggering hunger and cravings. Protein is like logs. It gives you more sustained energy than carbs. But the best fuel source is fat. It's your body's coal—the steadiest, longest-lasting source of energy. And the only way to get your body to burn fat, aside from going on a no-food or low-food fast, is to eat a satisfying, nutrient-rich ketogenic diet. My keto diet's ratio of high fat to low carbs forces your body to dip into its stubborn fat stores for fuel—a physiological shift that's as broadly beneficial as exercise in terms of the array of effects it can have on your body.

Sadly, we're in desperate need of dietary rescue. In the 1960s, doctors began recommending a low-fat diet as the path to better health, and by the 1990s the USDA conveyed this message to the public in the form of a food pyramid: A healthy diet, the pyramid showed, should be built upon a solid foundation of bread, cereal, rice, and pasta—and as little fat as possible. Based on that fat-is-bad mentality, we swapped out all the healthy fats that had fueled people's bodies and brains for thousands of years—things like bone broth and grass-fed meats and avocados and coconuts—for carbs, carbs, and more carbs. For proof, go to your local grocery store and walk around the aisles. What do you see? At least half the store is likely to be packaged carbs. Cereal, crackers, pasta, sauces, salad dressing, bread, cookies, candy, soda. Those jam-packed shelves are the epicenter of the obesity epidemic, the place where most of our nation's current health problems were born.

Diabetes is a prime example. It's one of the top ten most common health conditions in the United States. Almost 10 percent of people[1]—that's more than 30 million nationwide—now have the illness, putting them at risk of all sorts of other serious health problems, like heart disease, stroke, kidney failure, vision loss, and premature death. More than half of limb amputations in the United States are attributable to diabetes. It literally causes loss of life and limb. And there are 84 million more people with blood sugar numbers that put them in the prediabetic range—people who are teetering on the brink of developing the full-blown version of the disease. That boggles my mind. In 1958, just 1.5

million people were diagnosed with diabetes.[2] Now, more than 100 million adults in the United States are living with prediabetes or diabetes—and facing all the serious health consequences that occur when your body is overrun by glucose.

Deb McFeely, of San Diego, was almost one of them. Her doctor told her, at age fifty-nine, that her blood sugar was high. Not long after receiving that unsettling news, she heard about Keto360, a program I created with my colleagues Jordan Rubin, Dr. Jason Olafsson, and Dr. Isaac Jones, which forms the foundation of the comprehensive approach I've laid out in this book. Worried about her health, she decided to give the diet a try.

In the first month Deb lost thirteen pounds, along with *eight inches* of body fat—five from around her waist, an inch from each thigh, and half an inch from each of her arms. "I've dieted off and on most of my adult life, and this is hands down the most effective and easiest thing I've ever done," she says. "The diet is so filling I sometimes have to remind myself to eat, and I rarely crave sugar anymore. I'm sleeping better, too. I used to wake up a lot during the night and feel exhausted all day. Now I have this deep, restful sleep so my energy is higher."

But the real moment of truth came when Deb went back to her doctor. "He told me I had completely reversed my blood sugar. My numbers were back in the normal range," she recalls. "It was a really great moment. I'm getting older and my health is important to me. But I wasn't sure I could do anything to change my blood sugar. Getting off sugar and bread and eating more vegetables and healthy fat has restored my health. And I'm back in the skinny jeans I wore five years ago. This isn't just a diet. I see it as a recipe for living."

THE TOP SEVEN HEALTH PROBLEMS THE KETO DIET CAN HELP

I never get tired of hearing stories like Deb's. They remind me that I'm doing what I was meant to do—not just offering people a way to look good in their clothes but actually helping them heal the underlying problems that crop up because of our modern lifestyle. If you suffer from any number of common ailments—abnormal blood sugar, high cholesterol, hormonal issues, chronic inflammation, lack of energy, or difficulty concentrating, a key factor is likely your overconsumption of carbohydrates. If you've struggled for years to lose weight but never had long-term success, carbs are probably to blame as well. But more and more research is showing that by getting back to ancient nutrition, eating lots of healthy fats and tapping into the powerful state of ketosis, you give your body the opportunity to clear out toxins, reset hormones, fight a staggering array of diseases, and essentially cure itself.

Ketosis is beneficial for the following seven all-too-common health-related issues. If you're struggling with any one of them, my keto diet program is for you.

Diabetes. When we eat processed foods and refined sugar, they flood our bloodstream with glucose. It's not healthy to have too much sugar in the blood, so your body does its best to get rid of it; the pancreas swings into action and secretes insulin—the hormone that moves excess glucose out of the blood and into the liver, muscles, and body fat. But when most of your calories come from foods like pasta, bread, chips, and crackers, your pancreas is constantly churning out high levels of insulin. Over time, your cells adapt to the onslaught of insulin by reducing the number of insulin-sensitive receptor cells on their surface. They become insulin-resistant, a key contributor to diabetes and heart disease.

Think of it this way: Each cell is a house with a certain number of doors. Insulin is the only substance that can open the doors and let glucose into the house. When the body produces too much insulin, the "houses" respond by reducing the number of doors—which means insulin and glucose pile up outside, in the blood. When you have too much sugar in your bloodstream, it causes system-wide inflammation, wears away at your arteries and organs, and damages your whole body, making you old before your time. The pancreas doesn't know the number of doors has decreased, so it responds by producing *more* insulin to remove the excess blood sugar. That helps for a while. But at a certain point, the pancreas can't keep up with the increased demand. When that happens—when you have high blood sugar paired with insulin-resistant cells—you become a national statistic: You're diabetic.

KETO DIET VS. STANDARD DIET

Keto Diet: High Fat

Balances blood sugar
▼
Lipase releases triglycerides
▼
Fat goes to the liver
▼
Liver produces ketones for energy

Standard Diet: High Carb

Increases blood sugar
▼
Pancreas releases insulin
▼
Sugar enters the cells
▼
Cells use sugar for energy

Fortunately, clinical studies are proving that what happened to Deb is the norm: In a study published in the journal *Nutrition & Metabolism*, researchers from Duke University Medical Center and the Department of Veterans Affairs Medical Center put overweight people with type 2 diabetes on a ketogenic diet for sixteen weeks.[3] By the end, more than 80 percent of participants' glycemic control was so much better, they were able to reduce the dosage of their medications—and more than a third of participants discontinued their meds entirely. As researchers in Italy pointed out in a comprehensive review of the therapeutic uses of the ketogenic diet not long ago, when people with type 2 diabetes go on a ketogenic diet, "results have been nothing short of remarkable."[4]

Heart disease. Steering clear of raging blood sugar and out-of-control insulin is good for your heart as well. But there are additional ways the ketogenic diet protects your cardiovascular system. A 2013 study published in the *British Journal of Nutrition* found that those following a keto diet achieved better long-term body weight and cardiovascular risk factor management when compared with people assigned to a conventional low-fat diet.[5] The keto diet lowers cholesterol and triglycerides, while increasing the level of good HDL cholesterol—reducing common risk factors for heart attack and stroke.

KETO DIET BENEFITS

CAUSES WEIGHT LOSS (FAT)

HOW?
▶ Uses fat instead of sugar for fuel
▶ Lowers insulin so the body stores less fat
▶ Significantly reduces appetite

FIGHTS TYPE 2 DIABETES

HOW?
▶ Prevents excessive insulin release
▶ Creates normal blood sugar levels

FIGHTS HEART DISEASE

HOW?
▶ Lowers bad (LDL) cholesterol
▶ Lowers triglycerides
▶ Raises good (HDL) cholesterol

PROTECTS AGAINST CANCER

HOW?
▶ May "starve" cancer cells (high-sugar diets feed cancer cells)

FIGHTS NEUROLOGICAL DISORDERS

HOW?
▶ Improves mitochondrial function
▶ Yields a neuroprotective effect

IMPROVES LONGEVITY

HOW?
▶ Triggers fasting state linked to longevity gene
▶ Reduces inflammation, a driver of disease

Weight loss. Most people lose a significant amount of weight on my keto diet program—and do so quickly. In one study, eighty-three obese patients who weighed between 218 and 227 pounds were put on a ketogenic diet.[6] After eight weeks they'd lost, on average, twenty-two pounds—and after twenty-four weeks they'd lost as many as forty-two pounds. I saw even more astounding weight loss in my clinic, as have colleagues of mine who prescribe a keto diet in their functional medicine practices. When you're eating a satisfying diet that helps you burn body fat for fuel and reduce your levels of the fat-storage hormone, insulin, it's easy to lose weight and keep it off.

Epilepsy and seizure disorders. The ketogenic diet was discovered in the early 1920s, when several doctors around the country began looking at diet as a way to treat epilepsy.[7] They already knew that fasting was remarkably effective at reducing and even eliminating seizures. Fasting had been used since at least 2000 BC. It's mentioned in the Hippocratic Corpus, a collection of about sixty ancient Greek medical documents associated with the teachings of Hippocrates, the "father of medicine," and is recommended in the Bible for physical, mental, and spiritual health benefits.

But fasting obviously isn't feasible as a long-term treatment. So Dr. Russell Wilder at the Mayo Clinic and a group of MDs at Harvard began experimenting with diets to see if they could find a way to mimic fasting while allowing patients to eat—and came to the same conclusion: A very-low-carb, high-fat diet not only created the same biological state as fasting but also had the same beneficial effect on children with seizures. (Epilepsy is more common in young children and the elderly than in teens and adults.) Their behavior and cognition seemed to improve as well. In another early study of more than a thousand children at Johns Hopkins Hospital who were prescribed the diet, 52 percent attained complete seizure remission and 27 percent had a significant reduction.[8]

I've heard similar stories. When a neurologist recommended a ketogenic diet for Hayleigh, Eric Alber's ten-year-old daughter, who has intractable seizures due to a rare developmental disorder known as Smith-Magenis syndrome, Eric decided both he and his daughter should try my keto protocol. Prior to starting the diet, Hayleigh was having at least one small seizure every day and a grand mal seizure every two or three weeks—and antiseizure medications only made Hayleigh's underlying syndrome worse.

"The first month on the keto diet, Hayleigh had zero seizures, not even the tiny ones she'd been having daily. She's had some episodes since, but I think they happened when she wasn't in ketosis. She is also functioning better cognitively. She's mellower, more talkative, and more jovial—and she's sleeping about six or seven solid hours a night. That was unheard of before. It has helped both of us feel better."

In fact, Eric dropped from 214 to 190 pounds and a size 40 to a size 34 pant—and the stubborn love handles and belly he could never get rid of are almost gone. "I did this diet for Hayleigh," he says, "but it has really saved me, too."

Other neurological disorders. A *European Journal of Clinical Nutrition* study pointed to emerging data suggesting that the ketogenic diet can be helpful for treating numerous neurological disorders, including headaches, head injuries like concussions, Parkinson's, sleep disorders, brain cancer, autism, and multiple sclerosis.[9] A sample of the promising research:

- Studies have found the diet may improve the cognitive functioning of Alzheimer's patients.[10]
- In patients with Parkinson's, the severity of symptoms decreased by 43 percent after a month on the ketogenic diet.[11]
- Case studies reported in the medical journal *Frontiers in Pediatrics* found improved learning abilities and social skills in autistic children following a ketogenic diet.[12]

Despite their different symptoms, most neurological diseases share a common underlying abnormality: Sufferers' brain cells show deficient or defective energy production. And that's where my keto diet program can be extremely beneficial. Ketones, the fuel you burn when you're in ketosis, easily cross the blood-brain barrier and increase the number and functioning of mitochondria, the brain cells' "energy factories"—especially in the hippocampus, a brain region important for learning and memory.

In people with age-related brain diseases, like Alzheimer's and dementia, symptoms like memory loss are caused by degeneration of cells in the hippocampus. Because ketosis helps mitochondria churn out more energy, it protects vulnerable brain cells from disease-related problems that would ordinarily kill them.

In addition, ketones are a more efficient fuel than glucose for the

WHAT ARE KETONES?

Ketosis occurs when the liver breaks down fat into fatty acids—a process called beta-oxidation. The body then breaks down these fatty acids into ketones, which you can burn as fuel.

WHY ARE KETONES IMPORTANT?

 Once ketone levels in the blood rise to a certain point, then you've offically entered the metabolism-boosting state of ketosis.

 When your body stays fueled with circulating ketones, your metabolism is altered in a way that turns you into a "fat-burning machine."

Many experts consider burning ketones to be a "cleaner" way to stay energized compared to running on carbs and sugar. Burning ketones has been shown to cause less oxidative damage to cells, which in turn helps them create more energy.

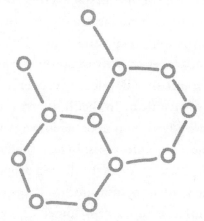

brain, providing more energy per unit of oxygen used, and they inhibit the production of damaging free radicals, unpaired electrons that are a normal by-product of cellular metabolism but can harm cells and their DNA and are a hallmark of aging and brain degeneration. As a result, the ketogenic diet holds promise not just for reducing symptoms and slowing the progression of devastating neurological disorders but also for bolstering the cognitive performance of healthy people and shielding their brains from age-related decline.

Cancer. I have no way of knowing for certain what ultimately caused my mom's second bout of cancer to retreat, but my medical instinct and understanding of how ketosis affects the biology of cancer cells tells me her keto-like diet had a lot to do with it. Studies suggest that ketogenic diets may starve cancer cells—and here's how: While healthy cells in our body are able to use fat for fuel, cancer cells seem to preferentially feed on glucose. A highly processed, inflammation-producing, low-nutrient, carb-heavy diet may fuel cancer cells, causing them to proliferate and spin out of control. Glucose is the juice cancer needs to survive and spread.

As long ago as 1987, researchers began reporting decreased tumor weight and improved strength and body weight in mice with colon cancer that were put on a ketogenic diet.[13] Animal studies since then have shown that ketogenic diets limit tumor growth and improve survival in a range of different types of cancer, including glioma (a cancer that affects the brain and spinal cord), colon cancer, gastric cancer, and prostate cancer.[14] At the same time, there's reason to believe that by helping you lose weight and reduce inflammation—both of which are factors in cancer growth and proliferation—following a keto diet can reduce your risk of developing cancer in the first place.

Inflammation. In the short term, inflammation is a good thing. It's your body's first line of defense against all sorts of harmful insults, from injuries to infections. In fact, the swelling, redness, and pain of an inflammatory response are all vital proponents of the healing process.

When inflammation goes on too long, however, it's dangerous. When inflammatory cells linger in your blood vessels, for instance, they promote the buildup of dangerous plaque, which ratchets up the risk of heart attack and stroke. Chronic inflammation can also play a role in Alzheimer's, inflammatory bowel disease, arthritis, cancer, psoriasis, lung disease, depression, and gum disease—and even impede weight loss by impairing hunger and satiety signals and slowing metabolism.

But here's the great news: Evidence is building that the ketogenic diet can be a powerful inflammation fighter. If you think of inflammation as an internal fire, ketosis tames the flames by producing fewer free radicals than when your body is metabolizing carbohydrates—and free radicals fuel inflammation. At the same time, when the liver turns fatty acids into ketones, it elevates levels of adenosine, a substance that is one of the body's best natural anti-inflammatories. And my keto diet program contains tons of anti-inflammatory foods, from berries to herbs, designed to make the most of this natural beneficial effect of ketosis and restore your body to a state of wellness.

KETO YOUR WAY TO A LONGER, HEALTHIER LIFE

When Kristy Marchand, fifty-eight, a retired army veteran in Bullhead City, Arizona, stepped on the scale in her doctor's office, she almost couldn't believe her eyes. At five feet eight inches tall, she weighed 245 pounds. According to the BMI chart, she was obese. Kristy had been active her whole life and never had to worry about her weight. Then, while taking steroids for a tumor in her eye that her doctor thought was cancer (it wasn't), she put on weight—and the extra pounds, along with the uncertainty about her health, made her depressed. So she did what many of us do—she turned to carbs for comfort.

By the time she stepped on the scale at the doctor's office, Kristy had developed arthritis in her neck, lower back, and knees that made every movement painful. "I was absolutely miserable, so I talked my husband into doing the ketogenic diet with me," she says. After four months on my keto diet protocol, Kristy had lost thirty-six pounds and her husband had lost forty—and the pain from her arthritis is a distant memory, probably because the high-fat, low-carb approach reduced her inflammation. "We feel so much better," she says. "We've realized that this eating plan can help keep us healthy for the rest of our lives."

There's every reason to believe that my keto diet program can help *all* of us age more healthfully. After all, as I've mentioned, it was discovered because it puts the body into ketosis, just like fasting. And fasting is one of the most effective ways to increase longevity. Studies have shown that reducing calorie consumption by 30 to 40 percent extends life span by a third or more in many animals[15]—and there's also data showing that limiting food intake can keep you healthier as you age. It not only adds years to your life; it adds life to your years. Fasting mice, for instance, have higher levels of BDNF (brain-derived neurotrophic factor), a protein that prevents stressed brain cells from dying. And it escalates autophagy, the body's system for getting rid of damaged molecules, including ones that are tied to neurological diseases like Alzheimer's and Parkinson's.

Indeed, studies have shown that intermittent fasting is associated with greater life span and health span. When University of Florida researchers put nineteen people on an alternate-day fasting program (in which they ate normally one day, then consumed fewer than 500 calories the next) for just three weeks, the participants' cells began making more copies of the SIRT3 gene,[16] one of several longevity genes that prevent free radical production and improve cells' ability to repair mutations.

Evidence is emerging that the ketogenic diet mimics fasting's longevity benefits. A 2017 study at the Buck Institute for Research on Aging found that mice fed a ketogenic diet lived significantly longer, on average, than those fed a control diet—and older mice on the ketogenic diet were remarkably spry, with better motor function, muscle mass, and memory.[17] No similar head-to-head study has ever been done in humans, nor will it, since people live far longer and can't be trusted to stick to a strictly controlled diet for years on end. But a study in the renowned medical journal *The Lancet* that looked at more than 135,000 adults in eighteen countries found that a high-carb diet was associated with a higher risk of mortality, whereas a high-fat diet was associated with lower death rates.[18]

The potential of ketosis to protect and promote health is staggering. That's why I believe so wholeheartedly in my keto diet program. And it's my hope that by understanding how this plan can help you look and feel better in the here and now, reduce your risk for many of the diseases that often strike with age, and add healthy, vibrant years to your life, you'll recognize the promise and power of my keto diet, too.

CHAPTER 3

How to Kick-Start Ketosis

The Art of Macro Manipulation and the Eight Critical Keto Strategies

Several years into my practice, a new patient came to see me. Dave was a friendly guy, a former high school football player, who had put on a few pounds every year since he'd stopped playing. By the time he wound up in my office, he was in his thirties and twenty-five pounds overweight—and his health was suffering. His blood sugar levels put him in the prediabetes zone, and he was taking medication to keep his blood pressure and cholesterol under control. He told me he had recently started on a ketogenic diet to try to get his health under control—and although he'd lost a few pounds, he wasn't feeling great. "Here's the problem, Doc," he said. "My joints hurt. I'm tired and sluggish. My skin is breaking out like when I was in high school. I've heard great things about this diet but I can't figure out what's going on. Can you help me?"

I told Dave I was glad he'd found the ketogenic diet and explained that many of my patients had incredible success with the approach. "But," I said, "there's a right and a wrong way to go keto—and without some guidance, it's easy to run into problems." I told Dave he had a classic case of the keto flu, a condition that sometimes develops when people's bodies are shifting from burning sugar to burning fat and adjusting to ketosis. But keto flu isn't inevitable, I explained—and it's actually unlikely if you approach the diet the right way. "Tell me what you're eating on a daily basis," I said to Dave, "and I bet we can sort this out."

Dave outlined his usual day: Breakfast was coffee with bacon fried in butter. Lunch was usually a bacon, egg, and cheese wrap in a grain-free tortilla. Dinner was a nonorganic burger topped with—you guessed it—bacon and cheese. I put my hand on his shoulder and smiled. "This is going to be easy to fix," I promised him, then gave him some suggestions for getting his keto program on track so he'd feel healthy and maximize his weight loss.

First, I suggested he substitute beef bacon for pork bacon (pork is often saturated with toxins and is more likely to carry parasites)—and limit the beef bacon to once a day. In place of bacon, I told him to start his day with a hearty, wholesome keto smoothie made from avocado, coconut milk, collagen powder, and spinach. Since the healthiest way to go keto is to consume a wide variety of antioxidants and nutrients, I suggested he have a massive lunchtime salad of nutritious greens topped with avocado, organic, free-range chicken breast, and olive oil. And for dinner I recommended a grass-fed, organic burger patty, to avoid the hormones and toxins of conventional beef, with a heaping side of oven-roasted veggies topped with ghee, a type of butter that contains fat-soluble vitamins and healthy fatty acids and can build stronger bones and enhance weight loss. I wrote it all down for him and asked him to come back in six weeks.

By the time I saw Dave again, he wasn't the same guy. He'd lost twenty pounds and looked trim and fit. His skin had cleared up and his energy was at an all-time high. His blood pressure and cholesterol had returned to normal, so he was able to get off his medications, and his blood glucose was back in a safe, healthy range—so he'd headed off the risk of diabetes, too. Not long after that visit, I heard he'd started doing half Ironman triathlons. I ran into him at a race years later, and the guy still looked incredible.

Over the past decade or so I've seen hundreds of Daves—people who are sincerely searching for a way to turn their health around and are ready to commit to the lifestyle changes that will make it happen, but who make some classic mistakes. They need solid, science-based guidance on how to implement changes in the safest, most effective way possible. I've made it my mission to provide that guidance. That's what my keto diet program is all about.

UNDERSTANDING MACRO MANIPULATION AND THE KETO FLU

Dave's story brings up a common hazard for people who wing it on the ketogenic diet. He read that keto was a high-fat approach to weight loss and built a diet around the fatty foods he loved to eat: bacon and butter. The trouble is, pork bacon and conventional butter aren't nearly as nutrient-rich as many other high-fat choices. By eating less nutritious sources of fat, Dave inadvertently increased the likelihood that he'd develop the keto flu. There's an art to macro manipulation, and in the keto diet I've carefully chosen the most wholesome types of fat, along with an array of nutritional ingredients that bolster energy and mental clarity, reduce stress (yes, food can help), and promote healing, to fully support your body as it goes into ketosis.

I'll explain more about those specific food choices in a minute. But first I want to expand on the keto flu and why it happens, because poor nutrition is just one of several reasons people experience symptoms shortly after starting the diet.

Entering ketosis transforms you from a sugar burner to a fat burner. There honestly aren't many other metabolic changes you could make that would be *better* for your health. But if you've consumed carbs your whole life, as most of us have, your body has never been anywhere near ketosis. So it's not uncommon to experience physical symptoms, like fatigue, headaches, nausea, and constipation during this process—hence, the keto flu.

In addition, if you've been eating a typical American diet, there's a good chance you're addicted to carbs and sugar—and as with any sub-stance you're hooked on, including tobacco or alcohol, it's common to feel withdrawal symptoms when you first break the habit. The com-parison between sugar and addictive substances isn't just theoretical, by the way. The medical signs of substance abuse are cravings, continued use despite negative consequences, failed attempts to quit, and withdrawal symptoms. Sound familiar? Nearly every sugar or carb addict I've ever worked with would say they've experienced these—and there's a good scientific explanation for why.

Research shows that sweets and high-carb foods affect the brain's reward system in much the same way that cocaine and nicotine do.[1] When this brain region is activated, it releases dopamine, a neurotransmitter associated with pleasure. The pattern is unconscious and uncontrollable. Every bite of sugar triggers a hit of dopamine, which makes you want more; when you stop the sugar-dopamine cycle by cutting out carbs, it sparks intense cravings. In fact, sugar cravings are the number one reason my patients say they can't stick to their diets.

Given the evidence that sugar is addicting, it's not surprising that the symptoms of keto flu are similar to those of withdrawal from other drugs: headaches, fatigue, brain fog, moodiness—symptoms that aren't dangerous but can make it hard to stick with the diet and lead some people to give up before they've had a chance to experience its benefits. But if you understand *why* those symptoms are occurring—that they're a sign you're breaking free of your longtime enslavement to carbs, including the energy highs and lows and the aggravating sugar cravings, and putting yourself on a cleaner, more wholesome path—the keto flu may be easier to cope with and less likely to derail your efforts.

Symptoms typically go away on their own within a few weeks, once you get through sugar withdrawal and your system adjusts to using ketones—the end products of ketosis that your body actually uses as fuel—in place of glucose. But by following my keto diet program, you can minimize the intensity of the keto flu or avoid it entirely. Over the years, I've identified the most nutritious foods that synergistically support the keto diet and can increase the likelihood that you'll breeze through ketosis feeling great.

Like many people who learn a little bit about the ketogenic diet online, Dave made a classic mistake. He focused solely on macronutrients—specifically, getting more fat and slashing carbs—instead of paying attention to the specific foods he was eating. By making bacon and butter the

KETO FLU REMEDIES

Side Effect	Remedies
Low energy	Caffeine and adaptogen herbs
Nausea	Peppermint and ginger oil
Hunger cravings	More healthy fat and bone broth
Brain fog	Rosemary oil and light exercise
Constipation	Water, probiotics, and magnesium
Difficulty sleeping	Lavender oil and collagen
Bad breath	Probiotics, green juice, and peppermint oil

main staples of his diet, he was missing out on all the vitamins, minerals, and antioxidants found in fat-rich foods like avocados, grass-fed beef, wild, fresh-caught salmon, nuts, and seeds—not to mention the veggies and herbs that are packed with nutrients and pair perfectly with healthy fat.

To be honest, people can run into similar problems on virtually any type of diet. I've known vegans and vegetarians who wouldn't go within a mile of a steak but still eat Cheetos. Here's the bottom line: While macros matter, the specific food choices you make are equally important. When you're changing your diet, you need to pay attention to the forest *and* the trees.

On my keto diet plan, the forest and the trees work in tandem to transform your overall health. For instance, recent research has shown that the healthy fat that forms the backbone of the approach actually promotes the absorption of micronutrients from the rest of the diet. In a 2017 study at Iowa State University, researchers had participants eat a big, healthy salad with a variety of veggies; when they tested study subjects' blood, they discovered that those who consumed more fat absorbed significantly higher quantities of seven vital nutrients, including vitamin K, two forms of vitamin E, and four different carotenoids[2]—substances that play a role in cancer prevention and vision protection. In fact, people who ate twice the amount of fat doubled their nutrient absorption.

Because my keto diet pairs rich sources of fat and protein with greens and herbs that are teeming with antioxidants and healthy phytochemicals, it has the ability to ease you through the transition to ketosis and amplify both your fat-burning potential and the amount of actual nourishment you take in with every single healthy bite. (For more guidance on how to start the keto diet, see my quick-start guide at www.draxe.com/keto-diet-kickstarter.)

THE EIGHT ESSENTIAL STRATEGIES TO SUPERCHARGE YOUR KETO EXPERIENCE

My keto diet program is a wholesome approach to eating, regardless of what your specific goals are—reducing blood sugar, resetting your hormones, losing weight, or just embracing a path to more robust good health overall. But I believe that if you understand why this approach is so healthy, you're more likely to make the commitment to stick with it. With that in mind, here are the eight critical elements of my approach that will help you avoid the keto flu and maximize the benefits of your keto journey:

Power up with plenty of superfats. Because the backbone of my keto diet program is healthy fat, you're going to be eating a lot more of it than you're used to. In order to stay in ketosis, you need to get about 70 to 80 percent of your daily calories from fat and round it out with 15 to 25 percent protein and 5 percent carbs. That can be tough to pull off at first, especially when you've been raised with a fat-is-bad mind-set. If you're hungry, it's tempting to grab your usual quick carbs or even protein. Instead, you need to find go-to foods that are high in fat, like avocados, nuts, and veggies with lots of ghee or real olive oil. Eating too few calories can contribute to cravings, moodiness, and fatigue. On my keto diet, you're going to meet superhealthy fats you might not ever have tried—including some powerhouse saturated fats that your diet has always been missing. MCTs, or medium-chain triglycerides, are saturated fatty acids that support brain function and healthy weight loss—and are largely absent from our modern Western diets. On my keto diet, you'll be eating lots of them. Coconut oil is a top source of

MCTs, for instance, and it's one of my favorites. MCTs bolster fat burning and weight reduction, help you feel full longer, and might even raise your metabolic rate, so you burn calories faster.[3]

Consume collagen, the most important ingredient you're probably missing. When you think about protein in your body, the tissue that usually comes to mind is muscle. But here's something most people don't know: Thirty percent of the protein in your body is made up of collagen. Ligaments, tendons, fascia, hair, nails, discs, bones, and skin—the largest organ in your body. Collagen is the tissue that holds your body together, like glue. It's the scaffolding that provides strength and structure and the substance that gives skin its springy elasticity. Gram for gram, type 1 collagen fibers, found in skin, tendons, organs, and bones, are stronger than steel. Unfortunately, your body's collagen production declines with age. That's why, as the years tick by, we develop sagging skin, wrinkles, and creaky, aching joints, as the cartilage that cushions the bones gradually wears away and isn't replaced. But it doesn't have to be that way. Our ancestors got plenty of collagen in their diets. They ate tendons, ligaments, and organ meats from animals and made broth from their bones. We get virtually none. And if you're looking to regenerate and heal your body, you absolutely need it. Collagen should make up 25 to 30 percent of the protein in your diet. Bone broth is the number one collagen food. You can make it yourself, buy it frozen, or purchase it in powder form and put it in your morning smoothie. (If you're using collagen powder, look for one that contains multiple sources of collagen, including types 1, 2, 3, 5, and 10.) You can also get collagen from the skin of wild fish, turkey, and chicken. And other foods support collagen production, including eggs, shiitake mushrooms, turmeric root, and fruits and veggies high in vitamin C, such as camu camu, citrus fruit, broccoli, and bell peppers. I emphasize collagen in my keto diet program because it's the most underappreciated nutrient out there, and it's vital for keeping the structure of your body strong, youthful, and free of age-related problems.

Veg out to alkalize your body. Even though the bulk of your calorie intake will be from fats, you should eat vegetables with every meal. They're important for a variety of reasons. The ultimate goal of my keto diet program is to help you feel better and get healthier, and in order to do that you need to alkalize your body. Here's what I mean by that. Every food falls into one of three categories—acidic, neutral, or alkaline—and produces those same conditions in your body. For example, eating too many processed carbs, which are acidic, can create chronic low-grade acidosis, which depletes your body of precious minerals like magnesium, calcium, and potassium, degrades bone health, increases inflammation, and sets the stage for chronic disease. Diets high in alkaline foods, on the other hand—like fresh vegetables, especially those that are green— promote an alkaline environment, which helps reduce inflammation, replenish your nutrient stores, and balance your body's pH levels (the measure of acidity in your system). Alkaline foods soothe the body from the inside out and create an environment in which healing can begin. Good alkaline food choices include dark leafy greens, avocados, mushrooms, radishes, artichokes, cucumbers, sprouts, broccoli, garlic, green beans, endive, and cabbage. Those veggies also contain lots of fiber, and, as a result, can help prevent symptoms like constipation and diarrhea that often occur during the transition to ketosis.

Herb up with adaptogens. We've all heard phrases like "kale is king" and "broccoli is best"; these veggies are powerhouses of the nutrition world that I encourage you to eat. But here's something you don't hear as often: Many herbs, like turmeric and cinnamon, are actually even more nutrient-dense than vegetables. They're nature's most potent medicine—and they're integral to my keto diet plan. They provide your body with important building blocks it needs to rejuvenate itself on a cellular level—and some of my favorite herbs are vital for curbing stress. You've undoubtedly heard that chronic stress can increase the hormone cortisol, a chemical that can damage the body in many ways. But one of cortisol's most dangerous effects is to promote fat storage. The deep belly fat that fuels metabolic problems is often the result of excess cortisol. Certain herbs called adaptogens tame this stress-related villain. Adaptogens are a unique category of healing plants that help stabilize your body, providing a potent antidote to stress. Herbs have been used for millennia by ancient systems of natural medicine, like traditional Chinese medicine and Ayurvedic medicine.

Now, cutting-edge science is catching up and revealing that herbs do indeed have the power to heal. I'll share more about the potent properties of herbs throughout the book, but here I want to highlight a handful that have the ability to keep cortisol in check and increase your overall energy. Following are seven adaptogenic herbs that can support and bolster your keto efforts by limiting the damaging effects of stress—and that have a host of other healing benefits as well:

■ Ashwagandha, an herb used commonly in Ayurvedic medicine, has been shown to reduce anxiety by relaxing the central nervous system.[4] It also may have anti-inflammatory effects; promote insulin sensitivity;[5] protect against cartilage damage and reduce pain in osteoarthritis;[6] and reduce the growth of breast, central nervous system, colon, and lung cancer cells.[7]

■ Holy basil, known in India as a powerful antiaging supplement, contains two phytochemicals that seem to lower blood corticosterone, another stress hormone. It helps protect organs and tissues from industrial pollutants and heavy metals and may fight chemical-induced lung, liver, oral, and skin cancers by increasing antioxidant activity and inducing cancer cell death.

■ Panax (or Asian) ginseng has been shown to exhibit a wide range of biological effects, including relieving and preventing mental fatigue and stress. In 2010, UK researchers reported that it improved some aspects of working memory and promoted a feeling of calm in study subjects doing mental arithmetic.[8] In Chinese medicine, it's used as a yang tonic (yang is the activating force in the yin-yang theory) to increase strength and stamina. It also has anti-inflammatory properties,[9] may bolster metabolism,[10] and may inhibit the growth of cancerous tumors, particularly those in the colon.[11]

■ Astragalus root helps beat stress by decreasing the release of some stress hormones and temporarily increasing others to allow the body to respond more effectively to stress.[12] It's also an immunity-boosting plant,[13] has heart-protective effects,[14] may slow tumor growth,[15] and has long been used for increasing strength and stamina by practitioners of Chinese medicine.

■ Licorice root can increase energy and endurance and has been shown to help the body more efficiently regulate cortisol,[16] thereby improving your stress response. It also has antiviral properties and is a natural pain reliever.[17]

■ Rhodiola provides a biological defense against stress by lowering cortisol. Researchers in Sweden also found that it helps people cope with stress-related fatigue by increasing the ability to concentrate.[18] It can also fight anxiety[19] and bolster weight loss by promoting the body's ability to burn belly fat.[20]

■ Cordyceps mushrooms, although not technically herbs or adaptogens, have notable impacts on cortisol as well. Studies have shown that they temporarily boost cortisol in response to stress, then trigger a large drop during nonstress periods, allowing the body to recover.[21] They also have important antitumor and immunity-enhancing properties. They contain complex sugars known as beta-glucans that may stop the growth and prevent the spread of cancer cells. When animals were fed beta-glucans, some cells of their immune system became more active.[22]

Hydrate. Dehydration makes every symptom of keto flu worse and can cause constipation, so it's vital to drink enough water—the equivalent of half your body weight in ounces. In other words, if you weigh 150 pounds, drink at least 75 ounces of water a day, in addition to the healthy green juices and bone broth smoothies you'll have as part of my keto diet program.

Embrace sea salt. Electrolytes like magnesium, potassium, and sodium can be lost at a higher rate during ketosis, as your kidneys flush them out—and electrolyte imbalances can contribute to headaches, weakness, and constipation. To combat this problem, I recommend adding sea salt to your meals. Sprinkle it on your morning eggs and your evening veggies. When purchasing salt, look for pink Himalayan salt and Celtic salt; they have the widest range of trace minerals that are beneficial for hydration.

Take advantage of caffeine. One common challenge of your body's transition to fat burning is a temporary lack of energy. Not everyone experiences it, but it can happen. When you're used to burning glucose, an easily accessible fuel that gives you quick, temporary bursts of energy, and you remove that option, it makes sense that you'd feel sluggish. Fortunately, caffeine is perfectly keto-friendly and is a great option for getting you through that low-energy phase. And guess what? A recent study shows that caffeine increases ketone production, especially when you consume it in the morning.[23] Check out my delicious Keto Coffee recipe on page 244.

Baby yourself. As your body is adjusting to ketosis, try not to overload it with an extra stressor like intense exercise. Get outdoors for a walk, do some yoga, take a barre class, or ride your bike to the store. But if you're feeling even mildly fatigued, hold off on high-intensity exercise until your body adjusts to your new regimen. At the same time, make sure you get plenty of sleep (ideally, seven to nine hours) and take breaks to relax during the day, since stress will exacerbate any symptoms you might be having.

HOW YOU CAN TELL YOU'RE IN KETOSIS

From a medical perspective, nutritional ketosis is diagnosed when the ketones in your blood reach a certain level. But measuring ketones in your blood, breath, or urine makes the approach less user-friendly, so I typically don't recommend it. I'd rather have you stick to my keto diet program than be put off by the need to assess your ketone levels. Besides, by paying attention to the way your body feels, you'll be able to tell when you're in ketosis.

Good signs of ketosis are weight loss, more sustained energy without the usual afternoon dips you typically experience when you're burning glucose for fuel, and reduced hunger and cravings. Appetite suppression is one of the most meaningful and obvious signs of ketosis. My patients who are used to battling the constant gnawing sensation of hunger when they're eating a carb-heavy diet say the feeling of being hunger-free while losing weight is one of the most rewarding and miraculous aspects of my keto diet plan.

Once you've reached a solid place with ketosis, you can start exercising normally. Regular physical activity is beneficial for everyone. In order to support your workouts, make sure you consume enough calories in general and especially get plenty of fat. If you're wiped out after a workout, it means you need to consider two possible solutions: consuming a bit more fuel and reducing the intensity of your routine. When you do high-intensity exercise, your body shifts to using glucose as fuel, regardless of whether you're in ketosis or not. So when you're on my thirty-day keto diet program, moderate-intensity exercise is the fat-burning, muscle-building sweet spot. Once you're on the Forever Keto Cycling Plan, you can schedule your workouts for the days when you're eating more carbs—an approach that allows you to train at a high intensity and continue to reap the benefits of ketosis.

I believe that arming you with information will set you up for success, but information alone isn't enough. My keto diet plan won't be fully effective unless you're willing to make some simple but significant changes. There's no magic bullet to transform your health. The only solution is to give up starvation diets and start living a lifestyle that will create long-term, sustainable wellness. You'll see results quickly with my keto diet program, but you shouldn't think of this program as temporary—something you're going to do until you turn around your blood sugar numbers or reach your goal weight. If you want to truly take charge of your health, you need to recommit every day, with every meal.

Small slips are going to happen. Beating yourself up for them is counterproductive and can make it more likely that you'll abandon the program. Just acknowledge that you've strayed from your plan and move on. Each meal is a new opportunity to make choices that align with your overall goals.

This isn't a sprint. It's not even a marathon. There is no finish line. By pledging yourself to this program, you're embracing a new way of eating that will set you up for a lifetime of wellness. The payoff is huge: a vibrant, disease-free future.

CHAPTER 4

A User's Guide to the Keto Diet

Foods to Eat, Foods to Limit, and Foods to Skip

There's a lot of talk about "hitting your macros" these days. That's just the latest lingo for getting the right amount of each of the three macronutrients—fat, protein, and carbs—in your daily diet. With the ketogenic diet, macros are important. For my thirty-day keto plan, I recommend a breakdown of 75 percent fat, 20 percent protein, and 5 percent carbs. But if you focus exclusively on those broad categories without looking at the specific foods you're consuming, you're going to miss out on some of the most powerful benefits of ketosis.

That's what makes my keto diet program different from any ketogenic approach you've seen. I've spent years searching for the highest-quality, most nutrient-dense sources of fat, protein, and carbs, so when you follow my keto plan you can be sure you're not only consuming the ultimate foods to put you into ketosis but also capitalizing on the serious, wide-ranging health benefits of burning fat for fuel, from tissue regeneration and collagen production to balancing hormones, including insulin, and healing your body. It's about using food not just as fuel but also as medicine. This thirty-day approach is designed to be a launchpad that sets you up for the longest, healthiest, most active life possible.

I began realizing early in my practice as a functional medicine doctor that not all foods are created equal. From 2010 to 2012, I had the opportunity (and honor) to help Olympic-level swimmers prepare for the 2012 London games. The swimmers were always asking things like, "What do I need to do to get a split second faster?" These highly trained athletes wanted to do everything in their power to eat the healthiest diet in the world—and they pushed me to find ways to help them do that. They didn't just train like Olympians. They wanted to eat like Olympians, too—and as I counseled them on their food choices, I came to an important realization: The rest of us should adopt an Olympic-level mind-set about diet, as well. You may not be competing for a gold medal, but your life has an important purpose, and your everyday actions are significant—whether you're raising children or taking care of aging parents or being there for friends and family. We should all eat like we're going for gold, so we have the energy, focus, vitality, and stamina to bring our A game to our loved ones, our jobs, our communities, and the world.

As you read through the sections in this chapter, I want you to think more like an Olympian. Rather than focusing on what you *can't* eat on my keto diet program, focus on what you *can* eat—and why those specific foods will provide the best, healthiest fuel for your body. That simple attitude tweak is surprisingly powerful. When researchers at the Yale University School of Medicine trained people to think about the positive consequences of healthy foods, something fascinating happened.[1] By focusing on the positive aspects of wholesome foods—their flavor, nutritional value, and health effects—participants started *craving* those foods more. And, over time, that subtle attitude shift helped study subjects make consistently better food choices in their daily lives. In other words, thinking optimistically about healthy foods actually helped them stick to a nutritious diet. The flipside works, too. Reminding yourself of all the negatives of the unhealthy foods—the fact that they clog your arteries, drain your energy, or cause you to store fat—can substantially reduce cravings for chips, cookies, candy, and soda. You can actually train your brain to want healthy food more and junk food less.

I've seen evidence of the power of patients' mind-sets to influence the outcome of the keto diet. When I go over the ketogenic food list, I can tell right away which people will succeed and which will fail.

Those who focus on what they *can* have are the ones who use the diet as a springboard for long-term health and wellness. So as you read through the food lists in this chapter, I'd like you to keep that winning idea firmly in mind. Instead of viewing healthy eating as a penance, see it as a privilege—something you *get to do* to be the best you can be.

FOODS YOU SHOULD ALWAYS EAT

Here's some great news: Once your body has adjusted to the health-promoting state of ketosis, you will experience more energy and less desire for junk food—a win-win. As you break your addiction to sugar, it will be easier to adhere to my keto diet plan. And the longer you stick with it, the more your body will crave healthy, nutritious foods in place of sugar-heavy, processed stuff. But to get to that point, you need to know exactly which foods to eat. Here's a breakdown of the keto diet food list—the healthiest way to nourish your body and brain. (For a simple list of the top twenty-five keto diet foods everyone should eat, visit www.draxe.com/keto-diet-food-lists.)

The fantastic fats

Fat is a critical part of every ketogenic recipe, because this powerhouse macronutrient is the secret ingredient that provides sustained energy and prevents hunger and cravings as well as weakness and fatigue. At the same time, it helps you absorb the nutrients in the other foods you consume. It literally supercharges your nutrient intake. And by getting up to 80 percent of your calories from fat and very few from carbs, you'll shift into fat-burning mode and begin to transform your health. Here are the three main types of fat you should have in your daily diet, along with keto-friendly foods that fall into each category.

Saturated fat: Controversial as this fat has been, the latest studies show it's not the bad guy it's been made out to be. Think about it: Forty percent of women's breast milk is made up of saturated fat.[2] It's essential for infants and remains essential throughout life. In fact, studies have shown that it's associated with a number of benefits, from better brain health in those with mild cognitive impairment[3] to a reduced risk of stroke[4] and higher levels of the good, HDL cholesterol,[5] which literally sweeps through your bloodstream, removing harmful LDL cholesterol from your arteries. Saturated fats form the foundation of each cell's membrane, the envelope that encloses and protects each cell and serves as a gatekeeper for substances moving in and out. Eating them actually helps your body burn fat and lose weight.

On my keto diet, you'll be eating these sources of saturated fat:

■ *Grass-fed butter*—Studies have shown that milk from grass-fed cows is significantly richer in fatty acids[6] and fat-soluble vitamins than the milk from cows on grain-based diets—which means the butter is, too. It's also higher in conjugated linoleic acid, a fatty acid that may be effective in reducing body fat, preventing cancer formation, alleviating inflammation, and lowering blood pressure.

■ *Ghee*—Similar to clarified butter, ghee is produced by heating butter to remove the milk solids and water, but it's simmered longer than regular clarified butter. It's packed with beneficial nutrients, like vitamins A, E, and K, which play a role in healthy vision and skin. Like grass-fed butter, it's also high in conjugated linoleic acid, as well as the short-chain fatty acid butyrate, which plays a role in gut health. What's more, it's lactose- and casein-free, so it's a good choice for those with milk allergies or lactose intolerance.

■ *Coconut oil*—Coconut oil is a great source of several types of important medium-chain fatty acids. One is lauric acid, which is found in breast milk. During digestion, lauric acid transforms into monolaurin, one of the most potent diet-related antimicrobials and bacteria fighters in the body, with the power to combat viral infections like the flu and common cold, yeast infections, cold sores, and genital herpes. Another is capric acid, which has healthy effects on the brain and contributes to the ketogenic diet's anticonvulsant effect, and the third is caprylic acid, which has antifungal effects that can keep your bladder, gut, and urethra functioning properly. Coconut oil also can reduce inflammation, improve thyroid function, boost your metabolism, and raise healthy (HDL) cholesterol. It has been shown to help heart disease patients lose excess body mass and whittle their waistlines, two factors that can protect your heart. You might have also heard that it raises unhealthy (LDL) cholesterol. But if you're eating an anti-inflammatory ketogenic diet, that probably doesn't matter. Sound crazy? Let me explain: Imagine your arteries are pipes in your home. If a pipe is damaged and springs a leak, you need to patch and repair the area. In your arteries, the patching is done with LDL cholesterol. That's why it's been known as the culprit in "clogging" arteries. But the *damage* is done by inflammation. In other words, the root cause of heart disease isn't cholesterol; it's inflammation.

■ *MCT oil*—MCT stands for "medium-chain triglycerides," a form of saturated fatty acid that has numerous health benefits, from improved cognitive function to better weight management. MCT oil is easy to digest and goes directly to your liver, where it has a "thermogenic effect" and actually cranks up your metabolism. Coconut oil is one great source of MCTs. Up to 65 percent of the fatty acids in coconut oil are MCTs, mostly lauric acid, one of four types of MCTs. But recently more concentrated oil that is made up almost entirely of MCTs has become popular. The advantage of concentrated MCT oil is that it contains all four different kinds of MCTs—and that may be important for your health. In studies, MCT oil has been shown to help with weight loss, improve heart health, bolster energy and mood, support digestion and nutrient absorption, and even help balance the bacteria in your gut that helps keep you healthy. Because of our fear of fat, these healthy oils are probably missing from your diet. It's time to add them back in. In addition to coconut oil, MCTs are found in palm oil and in small quantities in butter, cheeses (the best ones come from grass-fed cows), whole cream, and full-fat yogurt; while I want you to avoid dairy on my strict thirty-day keto diet plan, you can add small amounts back in once you're in keto cycling mode.

■ *Grass-fed beef*—According to a study at California State University's College of Agriculture, grass-fed beef includes significantly more omega-3 fatty acids and more conjugated linoleic acid (CLA) than grain-fed beef.[7] Along with grass-fed butter, grass-fed beef is a top source of CLA, a powerful polyunsaturated fatty acid that can fight cancer, reduce the risk of heart disease, prevent weight gain, and build muscle. In addition, farmers are less likely to use hormones and antibiotics on grass-fed cows. And here's another bonus: Grass-fed beef production actually benefits the environment by decreasing greenhouse gas emission, increasing biodiversity of pasture ecosystems, and improving the quality of runoff water from pastures.

■ *Cage-free eggs*—Eggs are one of the healthiest sources of protein around—and great sources of healthy fat. Although yolk-free recipes are popular, if you don't eat the yolk you're missing out on many of the vital nutrients in eggs. Yolks are an amazing source of choline, a nutrient that's important for liver and nerve function, muscle movement, and brain development, as well as vitamins E, D, K, and A; folate; and vitamin B_{12}. Eggs reduce risk of heart disease, according to a 2018 study,[8] and contain nutrients that do everything from improve eye health and slow sun damage on your skin to bolster liver function and brain health.

Monounsaturated fat: The term "monounsaturated" comes from this fat's chemical structure. Each molecule of this fat has one unsaturated carbon bond, making it liquid at room temperature and more of a solid when chilled. Monounsaturated fatty acids, or MUFAs, can help prevent depression, according to a study of twelve thousand people, reduce your risk of heart disease,[9] and potentially even protect you from cancer. They're also associated with *lower* levels of body fat. At the same time, MUFAs improve insulin sensitivity, help your body use fat properly, and strengthen your bones. MUFAs have potent anti-inflammatory properties—one reason they're so healthy. Inflammation is the root cause of many diseases, so any food that reduces inflammation is one you need in your diet.

On my keto diet, you'll be eating these sources of monounsaturated fat:

■ *Avocados*—In my opinion, avocados should be ranked one of the top five healthiest foods on the planet. This warty green food is actually a fruit that's jam-packed with MUFAs, including oleic acid, which can improve memory and brain activity and promote the absorption of carotenoids, inflammation-lowering compounds that give certain fruits and vegetables their bright yellow, orange, and red color. They're also a great source of fat-soluble vitamins, such as A, E, and K, and water-soluble vitamins B and C—and they contain vital trace minerals, including magnesium, potassium, iron, and copper, plus loads of fiber.

■ *Olives and extra virgin olive oil*—Staples of the superhealthy Mediterranean diet, these foods have been widely consumed by some of the world's longest-lived populations for centuries. Extra virgin olive oil (EVOO) has been associated with reductions in inflammation, heart disease risk, depression, dementia, and obesity. One word of warning: It's common for "extra virgin olive oil" in most major grocery stores to be laced with GMO-containing canola oil—a modified oil that can actually pose a danger to your health. To ensure you're getting a quality product, look for the California Olive Oil Council seal on the label or a harvest date, a single country of origin, and an ingredient list that says only extra virgin olive oil.

■ *Nuts and seeds*—Almonds, walnuts, cashews, macadamias, sunflower seeds, pistachios, chestnuts, pumpkin seeds, and tahini are good sources of healthy fat. Almonds, peanuts, and cashews, for instance, are packed with MUFAs, so it's not surprising that they've been associated with healthy outcomes, like improved insulin sensitivity and reduced belly fat. It's best to opt for sprouted nuts and seeds when you can, because they're easier to digest. Also, nut butters can be healthy, but many are loaded with sugar, salt, and hydrogenated oils. Look for raw, organic nut butters with minimal ingredients to ensure you're getting the best quality. Chia seeds and flaxseeds are both high in fiber, so they promote healthy digestion. But they're slightly higher in carbs, so watch your intake.

Polyunsaturated fat: Like monounsaturated fat, polyunsaturated fatty acids, or PUFAs, are liquid at room temperature and solid when chilled. PUFAs have numerous health benefits. They can help reduce "bad" (LDL) cholesterol in your blood, and they contain nutrients that help develop and maintain the health of your body's cells. They also provide essential fats that your body needs but can't produce itself, like omega-3 and omega-6 fatty acids.

My keto diet includes these healthy sources of polyunsaturated fat:

- *Wild-caught salmon*—Wild-caught (but not farmed) salmon is one of the most nutritious foods on the planet. It's credited with everything from extending your life span to preventing heart attacks and cancer. Here's why: It contains one of the highest omega-3 contents of any food and is bursting with tons of other vitamins and minerals as well. For instance, one 4-ounce serving contains more than a day's worth of vitamin D. At the same time, its high omega-3 content promotes bone and joint health as well as brain and neurological repair and healthy skin. It even helps prevent cancer. Farmed salmon, on the other hand, is on my list of fish you should never eat, because it's contaminated with toxins.

- *Walnuts*—Ever notice that a walnut looks just like the human brain? According to ancient wisdom, that's no coincidence. Walnuts have been shown to improve learning and memory and help fight depression—not surprising, seeing as they contain one of the highest amounts of mood-boosting omega-3 fatty acids of any nut. There's preliminary evidence that they might protect against cancer—and they make a filling snack while providing you with compounds that burn belly fat.

- *Flax, chia, and hemp oil*—Flaxseeds have been consumed for at least six thousand years, making them one of the world's first cultivated superfoods. They're chock-full of anti-inflammatory omega-3s, along with antioxidant substances called lignans that help promote hormonal balance. Chia oil has a nutrient profile similar to that of flaxseeds, while hemp oil has an omega-6 fatty acid known as gamma-linolenic acid, which is a necessary building block for certain prostaglandins—hormone-like chemicals that help control inflammation and body temperature and play a role in sustaining the equilibrium of your body's basic physiological functions.

Know the Smoke Point of Oils

When oil is so hot it smokes, it begins to break down, producing harmful free radicals, compounds you don't want in your food. The oil will taste acrid, too. So it's important to familiarize yourself with the smoke point of oils. Avocado oil and ghee are good choices for high-temperature cooking. Likewise, coconut oil and animal fats, like beef tallow and schmaltz (rendered poultry fat), are good at medium temperatures. When you sear meat you want to heat it as quickly as possible, so you need to use an oil with a high smoke point. The same goes for stir-frying. For sautéing, use oils with a lower smoke point. Always choose unrefined versions of oils.

Cooking oil/fat	Smoke point °C	Smoke point °F	Best for...
Flaxseed oil	107	225	Drizzling, dressing
EVOO	160	320	Drizzling, sautéing
Butter	176	350	Drizzling, sautéing
Coconut oil	176	350	Drizzling, sautéing
Beef tallow	204	400	Sautéing
Ghee	232	450	Searing, stir-frying
Avocado oil	271	520	Searing, stir-frying

The Lowdown on Omega-3, 6, and 9 Fatty Acids

It's important to get the right balance of these fatty acids. The human body can't produce omega-3 or omega-6 fatty acids naturally, so they're known as "essential" fatty acids; we have to get them from food. Here's what you need to know about each type:

Omega-3: The most well-known, omega-3 fatty acid is an important element of cell membranes and can improve heart health and mental health and fight inflammation. There are three main types: eicosapentaenoic acid (EPA), which reduces inflammation and symptoms of depression; docosahexaenoic acid (DHA), which is vital for brain development and function; and alpha-linolenic acid (ALA), which is used for energy. The best sources of EPA and DHA are oily fish, like salmon and sardines. ALA is found in chia seeds, walnuts, and flaxseeds. Our modern diets contain too few omega-3s, so it's important to have at least two portions of oily fish every week. There is also a unique type of omega-3 called eicosatetraenoic acid (ETA). Found in caviar (fish roe), it's even more anti-inflammatory than EPA and DHA—and comes in supplement form as well.

Omega-6: Used mostly for energy, this fat can produce pro-inflammatory compounds, known as eicosanoids. The Western diet is high in omega-6-containing vegetable oils, like soybean and corn, and provides far more omega-6 than we need. The keto diet replaces those oils with clarified butter, ghee, or olive oil. Hempseeds are a nutritious source of omegas-3, 6, and 9—and, as I mentioned earlier, the type of omega-6 in hempseeds is called GLA, which is beneficial for supporting hormone balance.

Omega-9: Our bodies can produce this fatty acid, but it's good to consume some through food as well. It's found in olive oil, avocado oil, almonds, cashews, and walnuts.

The powerhouse proteins

Your organs, tissues, muscles, and hormones are all made from proteins. The protein you get in your diet is used by every part of the body to help it develop, grow, and function properly. It's particularly helpful on my keto diet program, because dietary protein promotes satiety, stabilizes your blood sugar levels, improves your ability to learn and concentrate, bolsters energy, and supports the growth of healthy muscles and bones. Top sources of protein in my keto diet are:

- *Grass-fed meat*—Grass-fed beef is one of the best sources of protein—and it's rich in vitamins A and E, powerful antioxidants. But grass-fed lamb, goat, veal, and venison are also great options.
- *Wild-caught fish*—Add these delicious and protein-packed fish to your diet: tuna, trout, anchovies, bass, flounder, mackerel, salmon, and sardines. Each contains a variety of vitamins and minerals that bolster health.
- *Organic poultry*—Turkey, chicken, quail, pheasant, hen, goose, and duck are all good protein options that contain a variety of other

nutrients. Chicken, for instance, is a great source of B vitamins, like niacin and B_6, which are important for lowering your risk of cardiovascular disease, treating diabetes, supporting brain health, and lowering LDL cholesterol. Opt for fattier versions. For example, chicken thighs and legs are preferable to chicken breasts—and eat the skin, a super source of collagen. A compound that contributes to the formation of elastin and other substances, collagen helps maintain the youthful tone, texture, and appearance of your skin.

■ *Bone broth*—Bone broth made from beef, chicken, fish, and lamb was a staple for our ancestors, who used every part of an animal. But until recently it was almost absent from our modern diet. Simmering bones causes the bones and ligaments to release wonderful, healing compounds like collagen, proline, glycine, and glutamine that have the power to transform your health. Bone broth also contains minerals like calcium, magnesium, phosphorus, and sulfur in a form you can easily absorb. It's good for joints because it contains chondroitin and glucosamine, compounds that have been shown to reduce inflammation and help with arthritis and joint pain. It's healthy for the gut, too. It promotes the growth of good bacteria, fights sensitivities to wheat and dairy, and reduces inflammation in the digestive tract. And because it contains collagen, it preserves youthful skin. Finally, bone broth is a great way to obtain more glutathione, a substance that plays an important role in antioxidant defense, nutrient metabolism, and regulation of cell proliferation and death. If you don't want to make bone broth on your own, you can buy a protein powder made from bone broth that's packed with powerful amino acids.

■ *Cage-free eggs*—I talked about the many benefits of cage-free eggs earlier in the chapter, but they're also a super source of protein.

■ *Free-range organ meats*—We've gotten away from eating organ meats, often called glandulars, but liver is enormously healthy and full of an array of B vitamins, vitamin A, selenium, and folate. Liver, especially venison, beef, and chicken liver, is a superfood that is more nutrient-dense than kale and spinach. Misinformation has led people to believe that animals' livers contain toxins. But the liver actually metabolizes and helps the body excrete substances, including toxins.

Animal liver is not only free of toxic substances but it also gives your body key nutrients to support your own liver in detoxification. Other organ meats, like heart, have copious amounts of CoQ10, an antioxidant that is useful for preventing and treating certain diseases, like high blood pressure and heart disease, and kidney is loaded with selenium and other key nutrients that support adrenal and thyroid health. Spleen, pancreas, thyroid, thymus, and brain are all good options as well. In our culture, these healthy foods have fallen out of favor, but it's important to realize that they've been highly valued in traditional Chinese medicine for more than three thousand years. A basic tenet of TCM is that organ meats from animals support the same organs in your body. Indeed, organ meats optimize the function of your organs and promote their repair. Ancient cultures intuitively knew that organ meats were some of the most nutrient-rich foods on the planet—far higher in nutrients than the muscle meats we're used to eating. For instance, beef liver contains fifty times as much vitamin B_{12} as steak. The good news: If you have trouble eating organ meats, in spite of their profound benefits, you can now get their nutrients in supplement form.

■ *Protein powders and bars*—When you are on the go and eating keto, it can be crucial to have some healthy snacks and fast meals on hand. For protein powders I suggest you stay away from whey protein, which can cause blood-sugar spikes, as well as plant proteins, because they're difficult to digest. The most keto-friendly protein powders include bone broth protein, multicollagen protein, protein that comes from seeds like chia, and keto protein powders that combine healthy proteins and healthy fats. Also, a few types of bars, like bone broth protein bars, keto protein bars, and collagen protein bars, can be excellent keto snacks.

The most valuable (nonstarchy) veggies

You already know that foods like leafy greens and cruciferous vegetables are packed with nutrients, but when you consume them on my keto diet plan you're able to access more of their nutrition than ever before, because fat helps you absorb their healing nutrients. The veggies included in my keto diet program are all very low carb (yes, vegetables are carbohydrates). Eat as many of these powerhouse foods as you can.

- *Leafy greens*—Spinach, kale, romaine, chard, and arugula are the ones you probably already know about. But on the keto diet I want you to change it up and start eating things like dandelion greens, collards, watercress, mustard, fennel, broccoli rabe, and sprouts. Here's why: Each of these lesser-known greens contains important vitamins and minerals that can keep you healthy. Fennel, for instance, is high in calcium, magnesium, phosphorus, and vitamin K, so it's great for bone health. Collard greens are among the best sources of vitamin C and glutathione, which helps the liver cleanse and detoxify fat, boosts immune function, fights cancer, and protects the body from environmental toxins. And dandelion greens promote eye health and decrease water weight and bloat. They actually affect your body in a way that's similar to some weight-loss drugs, blocking the activity of a substance known as pancreatic lipase to help you excrete more body fat.
- *Cruciferous vegetables*—Load up on broccoli, cabbage, Brussels sprouts, and cauliflower. They're unique in that they possess a sulfur-containing compound called glucosinolate, which has been shown to have cancer-fighting properties and has been linked to everything from heart health to reduced inflammation. Cruciferous veggies are also high in vitamins A, C, and K as well as fiber.
- *Celery, cucumber, zucchini, chives, and leeks*—These veggies are all perfect keto foods because they're very low in carbs and high in nutrients.
- *Fresh herbs*—By now you know I'm a huge fan of herbs. In Chapter 3, I talked about adaptogenic herbs that help you fight stress and give your body the building blocks it needs to rejuvenate on a cellular level. Here I want to encourage you to use more seasonings like parsley, thyme, rosemary, sage, ginger, oregano, peppermint, and basil. They not only give food rich and varied flavor—I like to toss them in soups and salads or sprinkle some on top of meat and fish—but they also are packed with health benefits and have been used since ancient times for their

medicinal properties. Their power comes from protective polyphenols, plant compounds with potent antioxidant and anti-inflammatory effects. Preliminary evidence shows they can be helpful in fighting cancer, heart disease, and Alzheimer's.

■ *Veggies that are slightly higher in carbs*—Asparagus, mushrooms, bamboo shoots, bean sprouts, bell peppers, sugar snap peas, water chestnuts, radishes, jicama, green beans, wax beans, and tomatoes are great superfoods. They have more carbs than green leafy veggies, but the carb count per serving is still low—and they contain such a wide variety of nutrients that they're part of the foundation of my keto diet plan.

Fermented foods

You've undoubtedly heard the word "microbiome," which refers to the rich diversity of bacteria that live in your intestines. These microbes are vital for your health. They promote nutrient absorption and strengthen your immune system. Without them, you're at increased risk of developing digestive disorders, skin issues, food allergies, candida, and autoimmune diseases as well as reduced immunity, making you more likely to fall prey to seasonal colds and flus.

Probiotics are foods (and supplements) that support the growth of healthy bacteria in your gut—and chances are, your diet doesn't include enough of them. Throughout history, the human diet contained plenty of fresh foods from nutrient-rich soil that was teeming with healthy bacteria, as well as fermented foods, another source of beneficial microbes. Before the introduction of the refrigerator a century ago, fermentation was the only way to increase foods' shelf life. It not only preserves fruits, veggies, and dairy products but also promotes the growth of natural bacteria—and even elevates levels of some nutrients. Take sauerkraut, or fermented cabbage. It contains *twenty times* the amount of vitamin C as fresh cabbage and has far higher levels of lactobacilli, the beneficial bacteria that makes yogurt so healthy and lives in abundance on the surface of cabbage.

When you eat fermented foods, their healthful microbes take up residence in your intestines, where they serve as a first line of defense against harmful bacteria and toxins. To promote the growth of wholesome gut microorganisms, eat these probiotic foods regularly on the keto diet:

■ *Full-fat kefir*, a fermented beverage made from the milk of cows, goats, or sheep, is one of the most microbe-rich foods in the world, with up to thirty-four different strains of bacteria in each serving— and a staple of my diet. It makes a great base for smoothies. (There's a delicious kefir smoothie recipe on page 243.) Plain goat's milk and sheep's milk kefir is the best, but if it's easier for you to find the cow's milk version, that's acceptable, too. Coconut kefir is also a good option, especially for vegans. It's essentially a fermented version of coconut water and kefir grains and is available in most natural food stores' refrigerated section. Just avoid kefir with added sugar.

■ *Plain, full-fat yogurt* contains two superhealthy probiotics— lactobacillus and bifidobacterium—and often an array of others. The challenge with yogurt these days is finding varieties that are truly healthy. Many are loaded with sugar and made from milk from conventionally raised cows that were fed antibiotic-containing grains and corn, so they may contain traces of toxins and antibiotics. Opt for plain yogurt made from the milk of grass-fed animals. Goat's milk and sheep's milk yogurt are my preference, because they contain more nutrients and are less likely to cause digestive issues than cow's milk– based products.

■ *Sauerkraut* has been consumed for thousands of years, but these days much of the stuff that's available in stores isn't naturally fermented, so it doesn't contain the trove of valuable probiotics that the product is known for. You can still find the good stuff at natural food stores—or make your own. It's easy to make and delicious. Find my favorite recipe on page 274.

■ *Kimchi*, originally from South Korea, is similar to sauerkraut but far spicier. It is created by mixing Chinese cabbage with a variety of seasonings and spices like garlic, ginger, onion, sea salt, red pepper flakes, chili peppers, and fish sauce. The mixture ferments for three days to two weeks. You might need to develop a taste for it, but it's worth the effort. Research has found that kimchi lowers the risk of heart disease, diabetes, and metabolic syndrome. I'm a huge fan and like to put a spoonful on top of grass-fed barbecue beef or salmon.

■ *Natto* is made from fermented soybeans that contain *Bacillus subtilis*, a potent probiotic that has been shown to bolster the immune system, support cardiovascular health, and enhance digestion of vitamin K—which promotes bone density. It has a strong ammonia-like smell and an unusual stringy texture, so people either love it or hate it. But if you can develop a taste for it, the health benefits are worth it. Natto is one of the best plant-based sources of protein, so it's a great option for vegans and vegetarians. You can usually find natto at Asian markets or natural food stores.

■ *Miso*, a salty paste made from fermented soybeans, rice, or barley, has been a key ingredient in the Japanese diet for thousands of years. It's a great condiment to keep on hand because it can be used in a variety of recipes and offers some impressive benefits. Throughout history, it has been seen as a way to relieve fatigue, regulate digestion, decrease cholesterol and blood pressure, and prevent inflammation—effects that come from its high content of probiotics as well as numerous antioxidants and nutrients.

■ *Kvass* is a fermented beverage made from rye or barley that has Eastern European roots. It has a mild beer-like flavor but doesn't contain alcohol. This refreshing drink is a relative newcomer to the fermented food craze. If you haven't seen it at your local natural food store, chances are you will soon—and I encourage you to give it a try. In addition to its natural supply of probiotics, it has a wide range of nutrients, including vitamin B_{12} and the mineral manganese, which helps prevent osteoporosis and inflammation and is an excellent way to detoxify the liver.

THE BEST BEVERAGES

It's important to drink lots of water on the keto diet, because your body may get slightly dehydrated as you adjust to ketosis. You may even need more than the traditional eight 8-ounce glasses, especially if you're feeling low energy when you first start the plan. You also can have unsweetened tea or coffee in moderation, and you should be consuming at least 1 cup of bone broth or bone broth protein powder every day.

KETO DIET FOOD LIST

FOODS TO EAT ANYTIME	
HEALTHY FATS	▶ Grass-fed butter ▶ Ghee ▶ Coconut oil ▶ MCT oil ▶ Extra virgin olive oil ▶ Flax, chia, and hempseed oil
PROTEINS	▶ Grass-fed meat such as beef, lamb, goat, veal, and venison ▶ Organic poultry such as turkey, chicken, quail, pheasant, hen, goose, and duck ▶ Free-range organ meats such as liver ▶ Cage-free eggs including egg yolks ▶ Wild-caught fish including tuna, trout, anchovies, bass, flounder, mackerel, salmon, and sardines
NONSTARCHY VEGETABLES	▶ Leafy greens such as dandelion, beet, collard, mustard, turnip, arugula, broccoli rabe, endive, escarole, fennel, radicchio, romaine, sorrel, spinach, kale, and chard ▶ Cruciferous veggies such as broccoli, cabbage, brussels sprouts, and cauliflower ▶ Celery, cucumbers, zucchini, chives, leeks, and olives ▶ Fresh herbs ▶ Slightly higher-carb veggies such as asparagus, mushrooms, bamboo shoots, bean sprouts, bell peppers, sugar snap peas, water chestnuts, radishes, jicama, green beans, and tomatoes
FAT-BASED FRUIT	▶ Avocados
FERMENTED FOODS	▶ Kefir, yogurt, sauerkraut, kimchi, natto, miso, and kvass
NUTS AND SEEDS	▶ Nut butters and seed butters ▶ Chia seeds and flaxseeds ▶ Almonds, walnuts, cashews, sunflower seeds, pistacios, chestnuts, and pumpkin seeds
DRINKS	▶ Water ▶ Bone broth

FOODS YOU SHOULD EAT IN MODERATION

During my thirty-day keto diet, you are going to have to limit some foods you're used to consuming regularly, which can be tough at first. But as you get used to eating like an Olympian, you'll feel your body begin to function more efficiently, too. For most people, the trade-off is worth it. You can have up to one serving daily of these foods.

■ *Raw cheese*—As with everything, I advise buying cheese in its optimal state: unprocessed, raw, certified organic, and grass-fed. "Raw" means it hasn't been pasteurized. Pasteurization destroys bad bacteria, like listeria and salmonella—but also kills off probiotics and digestive enzymes. As a result, raw cheese is high in probiotics, including thermophillus, bifidus, bulgaricus, and acidophilus. Drinking raw milk can be slightly risky, because it can contain dangerous bacteria, but raw cheese is a different story. Cheese is essentially fermented milk, made by adding salt, bacteria, and enzymes to milk. As the product ages, it creates an acidic environment in which pathogens can't grow. As a result, raw cheese that has been aged for sixty days or longer is perfectly safe. Good options: cheese made from sheep's milk and buffalo mozzarella. Cheese that's not from cows is naturally high in calcium and vitamin B_2 as well as vitamin B_{12} and selenium—and it's easier on your digestive system and less inflammatory. As a general rule, hard cheeses have the least carbs while low-fat and soft cheeses have more.

■ *Medium-starchy vegetables*—Sweet peas, artichokes, pumpkin, spaghetti squash, okra, carrots, and beets each contain a variety of important nutrients and can be consumed in small amounts.

■ *Legumes and beans*—Kidney, lima, black and brown beans, chickpeas, lentils, and hummus contain healthy fiber and protein, but they're mostly starch, so stick with less than ¼ cup a day. (Find my tasty been-free Cauliflower Hummus recipe on page 277.)

■ *Fruit*—Blueberries, strawberries, blackberries, and raspberries are among the healthiest foods you can eat, but they contain a moderate amount of sugar, so you need to limit your consumption while on the strict keto plan.

KETO DIET FOOD LIST

FOODS TO EAT ONLY OCCASIONALLY

FULL-FAT DAIRY	▶ Full-fat sheep's milk ▶ Full-fat goat's milk ▶ Raw cheese
MEDIUM-STARCHY VEGGIES	▶ Sweet peas, artichokes, okra, carrots, and beets
BEANS/ LEGUMES	▶ Chickpeas, kidney, lima, black, and brown beans, lentils, and hummus
FRUIT	▶ Berries, including blueberries, strawberries, blackberries, and raspberries
CONDIMENTS	▶ No-sugar-added ketchup or salsa ▶ Sour cream ▶ Mustard and hot sauces ▶ Lemon or lime juice ▶ Salad dressing (ideal to make your own with vinegar, oil, and spices) ▶ Pickles ▶ Stevia (natural sweetener, zero calories and no sugar)
DRINKS	▶ Fresh vegetable juices ▶ Unsweetened coconut or almond milk ▶ Water with lemon or lime juice

■ *Condiments*—Check the labels of ketchup, salsa, sour cream, mustard, hot sauces, and salad dressing to make sure they contain less than 2 net grams of carbs per 2-tablespoon serving. Stevia and monk fruit will be your go-to sweeteners.

■ *Beverages*—Fresh vegetable juice and unsweetened coconut or almond milk are fine in moderation, and it's okay to add lemon or lime juice to one or two of your daily glasses of water.

FOODS YOU SHOULD NEVER EAT

Some of the following foods are too high in carbs. Others are just plain unhealthy, like sugar, and you should limit them regardless of the carb content. It can be tough at first to give up the sweet foods and snacks you're used to eating, but it helps to focus on the payoffs: increased energy, reduced risk of diseases, weight loss, and better health overall.

- *Any type of sugar*—That includes white, brown, cane, raw, and confectioners', as well as syrups, honey, agave, and anything containing fructose, glucose, maltose, dextrose, or lactose.
- *Any and all grains*—A single slice of bread can have 10 to 30 grams of carbs—enough to bust your keto efforts. Avoid wheat, oats, rice (including brown), quinoa, couscous, pasta, and pilaf, as well as corn and all products containing corn, including popcorn, polenta, and cornmeal. And no grain-based flour—or anything made with flour.
- *Most processed foods*—If it comes in a bag or box, you're best off avoiding it. Use canned foods sparingly, too. (For convenience's sake, you'll find a few scattered throughout my keto recipes.) Crackers, chips, pretzels, candy, cookies, cakes, pies, ice cream, pancakes, waffles, oatmeal, cereal, granola bars, meal replacements, canned soups, and anything containing artificial sweeteners should be banned from your kitchen.
- *Sweetened and caloric beverages*—Soda, beer, wine, liquor, sweetened teas or sugary coffee drinks, fruit juices, milk, and dairy replacement beverages, like soy and Lactaid, are high in sugar and will disrupt your efforts to stay in ketosis.
- *Cow's milk and low-fat dairy*—When you're on a strict ketogenic diet, you need to avoid cow's milk and low-fat dairy products. (Sheep's and goat's milk cheese, full-fat fermented kefir and yogurt, ghee, and grass-fed butter are all fine.) Milk, including full-fat milk, contains too many natural sugars to be keto-friendly. When you go into keto cycling mode, you can have small quantities of full-fat milk. But never use low-fat dairy products. The longtime dietary recommendation to opt for low-fat milk and other dairy products is just plain wrong. A 2016 study published in *Circulation* found that people with the highest consumption of full-fat dairy products had about a 50 percent lower risk of developing type 2 diabetes compared to people who ate less full-fat

dairy.[10] Another study that year of more than eighteen thousand women found that those who consumed more full-fat dairy were 8 percent less likely to be overweight or obese compared to those who ate low-fat dairy.[11] Full-fat dairy helps you feel full longer. Add the fact that low-fat and fat-free dairy products are usually chock-full of sugar, a risk factor for type 2 diabetes, heart disease, weight gain, and cancer, and the full-fat option is the best choice.

KETO DIET FOOD LIST

FOODS TO AVOID COMPLETELY

SUGAR	▶ White, brown, cane, raw, and confectioners' sugar ▶ Syrups such as maple, carob, corn, caramel, and fruit ▶ Honey and agave ▶ Any food made with ingredients such as fructose, glucose, maltose, dextrose, and lactose
GRAINS	▶ Wheat, oats, all rice (white, brown, and jasmine), quinoa, couscous, and pilaf ▶ Corn and all products containing corn, including popcorn, tortillas, grits, polenta, and cornmeal ▶ All types of products made with flour, including bread, bagels, rolls, muffins, and pasta
PROCESSED FOODS	▶ Crackers, chips, pretzels, etc. ▶ All types of candy ▶ All desserts (cookies, cakes, pies, ice cream, etc.) ▶ Pancakes, waffles, and other baked breakfast items ▶ Oatmeal and cereals ▶ Snack carbs, granola bars, and most protein bars or meal replacements ▶ Canned soups, boxed foods, and prepackaged meals ▶ Foods containing artificial ingredients such as artificial sweeteners (sucralose, aspartame, etc.), dyes, and flavors
SWEETENED & CALORIC BEVERAGES	▶ Soda ▶ Alcohol (beer, wine, liquor, etc.) ▶ Sweetened teas or coffee drinks ▶ Sweetened milk and dairy replacements such as cow's milk (and all low-fat dairy), soy, almond, and coconut milk, Lactaid, cream, half-and-half, etc. ▶ Sweetened fruit juices

ORGANIC VS. CONVENTIONAL? WILD-CAUGHT FISH VS. FARM-RAISED? HERE'S WHY IT MATTERS

One of the biggest mistakes people make when going on a ketogenic diet is to ignore the advice to consume organic and wild foods. I get it. You often pay more for these products. But if you are still consuming conventional meat and dairy products that are loaded with steroids, antibiotics, GMOs, and other chemicals, you may lose weight, but you'll miss out on the aspect of my keto diet program that I think is more important: the opportunity to heal your cells and organs, reset your hormones, and set yourself up for a healthy future.

My friend Jordan Rubin, who has written a number of books on healthy eating and studied naturopathic medicine for years, has a saying: "You can pay the farmer now or the pharmacy later." What he means is this: The very best sources of foods — organic produce, grass-fed organic meat, free-range eggs — might cost a little more than their conventional counterparts. But the cost savings in terms of your health couldn't be greater. When we purchase nonorganic food from the grocery store, we're likely eating produce or animal products teeming with toxic levels of hormones, antibiotics, and pesticides.

In a study published in the *Journal of Applied Nutrition*, organically and conventionally grown apples, pears, potatoes, wheat, and sweet corn were compared and analyzed for their mineral content over a two-year period.[12] The results were nothing short of jaw-dropping. The organic foods were:

- 63 percent higher in calcium
- 73 percent higher in iron
- 118 percent higher in magnesium
- 178 percent higher in molybdenum
- 91 percent higher in phosphorus
- 125 percent higher in potassium
- 60 percent higher in zinc

It's also better to purchase produce and meat from a farmers' market, so you know the food is as fresh as possible. Produce quickly loses its nutrient value after it's harvested—and the effect can be greater than you might think. Researchers at Penn State found that spinach lost 47 percent of its folate and carotenoids after only four days at room temperature and eight days in a refrigerator.[13] And a University of California at Davis study showed that veggies lose between 15 and 77 percent of their vitamin C within a week of getting picked.[14] Dozens of other nutrients begin diminishing during transport and storage of fresh fruits and vegetables because they are sensitive to air, light, and heat. Every day a food spends in transport, vital nutrients are lost forever. Add on a week in your fridge, and you see the problem. That kale you bought because it's jam-packed with nutrients may actually be delivering far less nutrition than you paid for.

Farmed fish is a problem, too. We all think of fish as healthy, but where it comes from is of paramount importance to our health. Farmed fish has high concentrations of chemicals, antibiotics, and pesticides. A study published in *Science* found that farm-raised salmon has eleven times higher levels of dioxin, a highly toxic chemical that lingers in your body for years, than wild-caught salmon.[15] Farmed fish also has lower levels of the nutrients, like omega-3 fatty acids, than wild-caught fish.

As you make your way through my keto diet program, you'll understand more and more why these choices matters so much. By providing your body with the highest-quality food, you'll begin to look and feel your very best. Choosing to eat organic is part and parcel of the Olympian mind-set. It's time to get your game face on and give your body the food it needs to thrive.

SWAP THIS...FOR THIS!

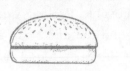

BUN

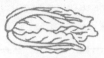

LETTUCE WRAP

CONVENTIONAL MILK

COCONUT MILK

BAKING FLOUR

ALMOND FLOUR

BEAN DIP

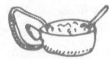

GUACAMOLE AND TAHINI

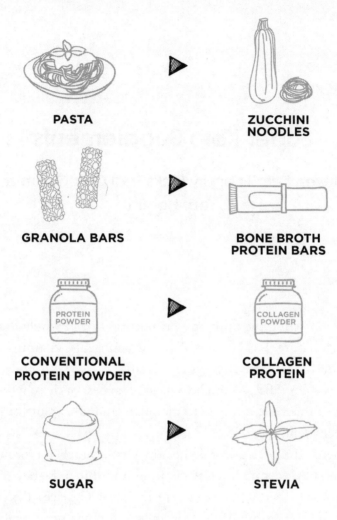

PASTA ▶ ZUCCHINI NOODLES

GRANOLA BARS ▶ BONE BROTH PROTEIN BARS

CONVENTIONAL PROTEIN POWDER ▶ COLLAGEN PROTEIN

SUGAR ▶ STEVIA

CHAPTER 5

Super Keto Supplements

Eleven Keto-Friendly Picks That Can Optimize Your Health

I believe in getting the bulk of your nutrition from whole foods that come from nature. Real food is alive with nutrients, vitamins, minerals, and antioxidants that act synergistically to give your body what it needs to ward off disease and heal itself. The best of these wholesome foods are at the heart of my keto diet plan, and no capsule or powder can replace them.

But here's the sad truth: The healthy foods we rely on for nutrients don't contain the same level of vitamins and minerals they did even fifty years ago, because modern agricultural practices designed to improve the size, growth rate, and pest resistance of vegetables and fruits have depleted the soil. A landmark study published in the *Journal of the American College of Nutrition* compared nutritional data from forty-three different vegetables and fruits from 1950 and 1999 and found declines in the amount of protein, calcium, phosphorus, iron, vitamin B_2, and vitamin C.[1] Don't get me wrong. Plant foods are still powerfully beneficial for your body; it's just that they don't supply the same level of nutrition they used to—which means supplementation is important.

On my keto diet program, supplements can also support your ability to get into ketosis—and stay there—and ensure that you're getting the most out of your eating plan. But you have to make sure you're choosing the right ones. Buying a generic protein powder off the shelf could backfire, for instance, because it might contain too many carbs and throw you out of ketosis. You need to select what I think of as "keto-optimized" supplements that have a healthy amount of fat from the most nutritious sources, along with an array of other vitamins and minerals.

These eleven supplements will round out and enhance my keto diet program. Some will ease your transition into ketosis. Others are inflammation fighters and antioxidants, so they'll bolster your overall health. And still others will power up your metabolism and increase your body's ability to burn fat. Consider the following list a comprehensive guide to the most effective keto supplements currently available. (For extra support and information on the top keto supplements and how to use them, go to www.draxe.com/keto-diet-supplements.)

EXOGENOUS KETONES

You already know that a ketogenic diet shifts your body out of carb-burning mode and turns it into a fat-burning machine. In that state, ketones are the fuel your body starts burning instead of glucose. The liver naturally produces "endogenous" (manufactured by the body) ketones once you're in ketosis, but exogenous ketones are supplements that can get you into ketosis almost instantly. Ketone supplements contain beta-hydroxybutyric acid, a substance that functions like a ketone, because it's converted easily into two true ketones—acetoacetate and acetone. Exogenous ketones efficiently and effectively raise blood ketone levels so you start burning fat for fuel right away.

Why would you take a ketone supplement if your body produces ketones naturally? Getting into ketosis through whole foods alone can take four to seven days—longer if you don't stick to the diet carefully. Taking a ketone supplement is an efficient way to elevate your blood level of ketones quickly so you start reaping the benefits of the approach sooner—and exogenous ketones create the same healthy environment in your body as natural ketosis does: They protect your brain, reduce inflammation, lower the risk of cancer, improve mental clarity—and slash your appetite, making it easier to lose weight. A study in the journal *Obesity* found that people who drank a keto supplement had significantly smaller appetites in the ensuing four hours than participants who consumed a sugary drink with the same number of calories.[2] By getting into ketosis more quickly, your body starts adjusting to burning ketones for fuel while you still have some carbohydrates in your system, which may protect you from experiencing symptoms of the keto flu.

How to use: If you have a powdered form, take 6 grams once or twice a day, with the first dose in the morning. If you have capsules, which are usually combined with synergistic ingredients, take 2 grams.

To get the most out of ketone supplements, look for ones that contain caffeine (if you can tolerate it), which can bolster your energy, as well as medium-chain triglycerides (superhealthy fats we talked about in Chapter 4) and bone broth. All these ingredients are part of my keto diet program because they support ketosis by promoting a healing, low-inflammation environment in your body. The best exogenous ketones also contain two other ingredients: bone broth oil, which is made from the nutrient-rich fat that rises to the top of homemade broth, and lipase, an enzyme that helps the body break down dietary fat so it's easier to digest.

KETO-OPTIMIZED PROTEIN POWDER

There are dozens of protein powders on the market, but most are made from whey, rice, or peas and will undermine your ability to get into ketosis, for one simple reason: They contain too many carbs and a too-high ratio of protein to fat. It's a common misconception that the ketogenic diet is a high-protein diet. It's not. It's a *high-fat, moderate-protein* diet. When you eat too much protein, your body converts some of it to glucose. Once that starts happening, you're no longer burning fat for fuel.

Keto-optimized protein, on the other hand, is one of the best things you can consume if you're looking for enhanced brainpower and sustained energy. It helps both your mind and your muscles function at their highest level and can be a powerful adjunct to the keto diet.

When you're buying a protein powder, look for one that has the word "keto" on the label—or check the nutrition contents to make sure it has keto-friendly ingredients. What to look for: Each serving should contain 10 to 15 grams of protein and 10 to 15 grams of fat, ideally from medium-chain triglycerides, or MCTs, and bone broth. That gives you more than twice the number of calories from fat as from protein, since fat has 9 calories per gram and protein has 4. Also, if you can tolerate caffeine, look for protein powders that contain a healthy source, like organic coffee fruit. Both caffeine and MCTs will bolster your body's ability to produce ketones, helping you get into ketosis and stay there.

How to use: Add 1 to 2 scoops daily (the equivalent of 20 to 40 grams of protein) to a glass of water or morning smoothie.

BONE BROTH PROTEIN POWDER

Protein powders made from bone broth contain all the same healthy ingredients as the bone broth you'd make yourself (but without the time commitment)—including large amounts of highly absorbable collagen. Bone broth protein can help your body flip the metabolic switch that allows you to stop burning glucose for fuel and enter the fat-burning zone. In Chapter 4, I explained that bone broth contains glucosamine and chondroitin—two substances that can reduce inflammation, support gut health, and protect your joints as you age. But I didn't mention that it also has hyaluronic acid, a lubricating substance that supports collagen and promotes beautiful skin, builds connective tissue, and repairs achy joints. In your skin, hyaluronic acid binds with water to help retain moisture. It does the same in your eyes, helping protect against dry eye, a painful condition that can develop with age. It also helps retain collagen and provides tissues with elasticity and flexibility. At the same time, the amino acids in bone broth support the growth of healthy bacteria in your gastrointestinal tract.

The key thing to look for to ensure that a bone broth supplement is keto-friendly is 11 grams of fat from both organic bone broth oil and medium-chain triglycerides.

How to use: Add 1 or 2 scoops daily to your favorite keto-friendly beverage.

COLLAGEN POWDER

You can take bone broth powder or collagen powder—or, for people who are looking for additional antiaging benefits for their skin, gut, and joints, I recommend taking both. Collagen is one of the most important substances missing from most people's daily diet—and we need it. It's the substance that holds your body together. It gives your skin its firmness and elasticity, your nails their strength, your joints the supple cushioning they need to move without pain, and your gut the microbes required to break down the nutrients in food and utilize them effectively. Up to 90 percent of our skin, hair, nails, ligaments, cartilage, and connective tissue is made up of collagen, as is a majority of our gut and arterial lining. Once you're thirty, your body's natural collagen production drops as much as 8 percent every year—and lifestyle factors, like eating a diet high in sugar, smoking, and getting too much sun exposure, accelerate the process. Getting extra collagen from a supplement will promote tissue healing and slow the aging process. It pairs well with the keto diet because it's a great source of protein with amino acids that are unlikely to be converted into sugar. To ensure your collagen powder is keto-friendly, make sure it has at least 3 grams of fat per serving from sources like MCTs or bone broth oil.

How to use: Add 1 or 2 scoops daily to your favorite keto-friendly beverage.

NOOTROPICS CAPSULES

Also known as "cognitive enhancers," nootropics are supplements that can improve your brain function, memory, creativity, and motivation.

They make an ideal adjunct for my keto diet program because they enhance the healthy effects ketosis has on your brain. I'll explain more about the many ways the keto diet supports brain health and bolsters cognition in Chapter 7. Taking nootropics when you're on my keto diet plan is like adding a turbocharger for your brain.

There are a wide variety of nootropics on the market. There are even prescription versions. As with all supplements, however, you need to take the right ones to support the effects of the keto diet. Look for the following powerful brain-boosting ingredients in a base of medium-chain triglycerides, one of the most nourishing sources of fat for your mind.

- *Citicoline*—This natural compound is found in every cell in your body, but it's particularly important for your brain—and you can't get it from most foods in the modern diet. The body can synthesize citicoline from choline-rich foods like eggs, beef, and seafood, but if you want to reap the full therapeutic benefits, you need to take a supplement that contains more of the compound than your body would normally provide. Citicoline raises the levels of several important neurotransmitters (the chemicals in your brain that help neurons communicate with one another), including dopamine, which strengthens motivation, productivity, and focus, and acetylcholine, a chemical that helps you learn and remember. It also increases blood flow to the brain, making you feel sharper and more energetic.

- *Ashwagandha*—This supplement is in a class of substances known as adaptogens, a group of compounds I told you about in Chapter 3. They're incredibly helpful in today's world, because they bring your body into balance. If your blood sugar is high, ashwagandha can lower it. If you have high cholesterol, ashwagandha will restore it to a healthier range. It has the same balancing effect on stress, anxiety, and depression. By affecting the neurotransmitters serotonin and GABA, which are known to play a role in mood and anxiety, ashwagandha can rebalance your brain. It has been shown to enhance memory, too. A study published in the *Journal of Dietary Supplements* found that ashwagandha not only enhances memory in people with mild cognitive impairment but also improves attention, information-processing speed, and mental skills.[3]

■ *Egg yolk extract*—Eggs are an excellent source of choline, a substance that reinforces brain function. Now nootropics companies have homed in on one particularly potent substance in egg yolks, phosphatidylcholine (PC), which has a number of promising brain benefits. PC is a source of choline, and it's found in abundance in the brain's cellular membranes. It not only promotes brain cell health by building and repairing cell membranes but also supports memory and cognition.

How to use: The formulation of these supplements varies by brand, so follow the standard dosage on the bottle.

ORGANIC POWDERED GREENS FOR ALKALIZING

One of the biggest challenges with any ketogenic diet is that you're eating more fat and meat than usual, both of which are acidic, so you need to load up on alkalizing foods. Veggies like wheatgrass, kale, spinach, celery, and seaweeds like spirulina and chlorella contain enzymes that maintain the brain and body's healthy pH balance—the balance between acidity and alkalinity. During keto, I like to add a supplement that contains organic, alkalizing greens, because it gives you all the superfood nutrients without any carbs.

Most of us never consider the acid/alkaline balance of our blood or tissues, but a proper pH balance is crucial to overall health, protecting us from the inside out. Modern diets high in simple sugars and sodium throw off the pH balance, tipping the scales toward damaging acidity. Restoring a healthy pH level, one that's slightly more alkaline than acidic, may prevent dangerous microbes and organisms from flourishing and minerals from being depleted, and may protect tissues and organs from damage and plaque from forming in the blood vessels.

As with any other keto supplement, you need to look for alkalizing greens that contain fat from MCTs, chia seeds, or flaxseeds. Healthy fat helps you absorb these nutrients and keeps you safely in ketosis. An alkalizing supplement can be especially helpful for women on my keto diet plan, because restoring alkalinity can promote hormonal balance and prevent some of the symptoms that women may be more likely to experience as they adjust to ketosis, like fatigue, constipation, anxiety, and hunger. It can also be helpful for athletes; alkalizing capsules can improve performance during intense exercise and enhance postworkout muscle recovery.

How to use: Add 1 or 2 scoops daily to your favorite keto-friendly beverage.

MULTIVITAMIN AND MINERAL CAPSULES

A good multivitamin is another way to help you get the nutrients you're missing from some of the healthy plant foods that aren't keto-friendly. Moreover, because the keto diet is high in fat, you can truly maximize your absorption of certain fat-soluble vitamins, like A, D, E, and K, so the multi you choose should contain healthy quantities of those nutrients in particular. Look for a multi that also contains several times more than the recommended value of B vitamins. Since you're not eating enriched bread and grains, which contain B vitamins, you want to ensure you're getting plenty of those nutrients—especially vitamin B_{12}—which are critical for maintaining your daily energy levels.

How to use: Formulations vary, so take the standard dosage recommended on the bottle.

PROBIOTIC CAPSULES

Probiotics have become popular for a good reason: They promote the growth of healthy intestinal bacteria—and a flourishing population of good bacteria in your gut can do everything from protect your brain to limit inflammation and bolster energy. Look for a probiotic supplement that contains soil-based microorganisms, like *Saccharomyces boulardii*,

Bacillus clausii, *Bacillus coagulans*, and *Bacillus subtilis*, which have been found to populate the gastrointestinal tracts of people who consume a healthy diet rich in fats and protein and low in carbohydrates. When you take a probiotic with those particular microorganisms, your gut will adapt to a keto lifestyle more quickly and you'll experience greater energy and health.

These spore-forming bacteria are able to seed your gut with beneficial microbes, so the protective bacteria will thrive and support healthy digestion and bowel function and strengthen immunity. Probiotics are particularly critical for people who struggle with bowel issues, but since the health of your microbiome plays a foundational role in determining your overall health, it makes sense for everyone on my keto program to take a keto-friendly probiotic.

How to use: Take 50 billion CFU one or two times a day.

DIGESTIVE ENZYME CAPSULES

There's an old saying in Ayurvedic medicine: "It's not what you eat; it's what you digest that's important." In other words, if you're consuming healthy foods but your body isn't able to break them down into their component parts so they can be used for cell regeneration, muscle growth, or brain health, what good are they? The way to ensure that you're actually able to use all the life-giving nutrients in the foods you'll be eating on my keto diet is to take a digestive enzyme supplement.

Again, it's important to take the right one. Most are geared toward digesting carbs and proteins. On my keto diet, you need one that's high in lipase, the primary fat-digesting enzyme, so it's optimized to help you get the greatest benefit out of every bite. A digestive enzyme can help you adjust to the keto diet, as well. When you're shifting from a low-fat, high-carb diet to a high-fat, low-carb approach, your body has to recalibrate its metabolic processes. Taking a digestive enzyme can ease that transition, helping your body adjust to ketosis—and can sometimes even make the difference between whether you'll succeed or fail on the diet.

How to use: Take the recommended dosage on the bottle with meals one to three times daily.

ADAPTOGEN CAPSULES OR EXTRACTS

As I've explained before, adaptogenic herbs and mushrooms, like ashwagandha, rhodiola, cordyceps, and reishi, can bolster brainpower, energy, and metabolism—benefits that complement and heighten the curative effects of my keto diet plan. These compounds help balance the body and have been used for centuries in ancient healing traditions. In the United States, we've largely overlooked these powerful, natural options for promoting overall health—a shame, since we stand to benefit the most by taking them, immersed as we are in a high-stress culture that promotes and encourages low-nutrient diets.

As you're adjusting to the keto diet, adaptogens can help you cope with stress, bolster your mood, reduce carb cravings, and smooth the transition into this new approach to food that flips the traditional Western diet paradigm on its head.

How to use: In capsule form, take 1,000 milligrams one to three times a day. If you're using an extract, follow the dosage instructions on the bottle.

MCT OIL

As I've mentioned before, medium-chain triglycerides (MCTs) are a form of saturated fatty acid that has truly incredible health benefits. Most of the supplements you take should contain MCTs, because they can help keep your body in ketosis. But taking an MCT supplement on its own can be beneficial as well. Medium-chain triglycerides can lower inflammation, improve cognitive function, help you maintain a healthy body weight, reduce stored body fat by revving up your metabolism, bolster energy and focus, improve your mood, fight bacterial infections, and absorb fat-soluble nutrients from foods. As if that's not enough, they're also the best fat for triggering your body to produce ketones. Supplements with coconut oil and palm oil are good options.

How to use: Take 1 tablespoon in a smoothie or other beverage (you can take it straight, too) one to three times every day.

THERMOGENIC HERBS

You know by now that I'm a big fan of herbs. They don't get nearly enough credit for how healthful they are—and thermogenic herbs, which bolster a healthy metabolism, boost energy, decrease inflammation, and reduce your risk of cancer, can be particularly beneficial on the keto diet. You can add these herbs to your favorite keto recipes and increase your intake that way. But if you want to add a controlled daily dose, they're all available in supplement form as well. Here are the herbs that will keep your metabolism high and nurture your keto efforts:

■ *Black and cayenne pepper*—These are such common kitchen staples you've probably never considered their health benefits—so prepare to have your mind blown. Black pepper is a superfood that can help prevent body fat accumulation and new fat cell formation. It can also elevate levels of good HDL cholesterol—and boost metabolism to promote weight loss. Likewise, cayenne pepper has been used as both food and medicine for at least nine thousand years. It can stimulate circulation, reduce your body's acidity, lower cholesterol, and stimulate saliva production, which can help with digestion. It's also packed with healthy ingredients, including capsaicin, which may reduce pain and help with headaches and arthritis, as well as vitamin C, vitamin B_6, vitamin E, potassium, manganese, and flavonoids, healthy compounds in fruits and vegetables that provide their vivid colors.

■ *Turmeric*—This herb is a functional food. The Mayo Clinic defines functional foods as "foods that have a potentially positive effect on health beyond basic nutrition."[4] Turmeric's benefits are well researched and grounded in ancient nutrition. Curcumin, the active ingredient in turmeric, is particularly known for its ability to control inflammation. The journal *Oncogene* published the results of a study that evaluated several anti-inflammatory compounds and found that aspirin and ibuprofen, the most common nonsteroidal anti-inflammatories, are the least effective, while curcumin is among the most.[5] That's a big deal, since inflammation is one root cause of most diseases, including cancer, Alzheimer's, arthritis, chronic pain, depression, and autoimmune illnesses. Indeed, research has found that curcumin is helpful for arthritis pain and cancer. In the words of Cancer Research UK: "A number of laboratory studies on cancer cells have shown that curcumin does have anticancer effects. It seems to be able to kill cancer cells and prevent more from growing. It has the best effects on breast cancer, bowel cancer, stomach cancer, and skin cancer cells."[6]

- *Ginger*—Another great anti-inflammatory, as well as an antioxidant, ginger is best known for its ability to treat nausea. It also lowers blood sugar (important as you're transitioning into ketosis), relieves joint and muscle pain by reducing inflammation, protects the brain against cognitive decline, and promotes healthy digestion.

- *Cinnamon*—This common spice has been used medicinally for thousands of years. It contains oils that reduce inflammation and fight cancer. Of twenty-six of the most popular herbs and medicinal spices, cinnamon contains the highest levels of antioxidants.[7] In other words, this herb packs a powerfully healthy punch. Cinnamon is also an effective anti-inflammatory and has been shown to reduce pain and relieve muscle soreness. At the same time, it can lower cholesterol, triglycerides, and blood pressure, so it protects heart health; it defends against cognitive decline by activating neuroprotective proteins that shield brain cells from damage; and it protects cells from DNA damage that can lead to cancer.

How to use: Sprinkle on food or in smoothies, or, in capsule form, take 250 to 500 milligrams of each type of thermogenic herb once or twice daily.

Supplements are designed to augment my already-healthy keto diet program—and they can be a game changer at helping you get into ketosis and stay there, as well as boosting your ability to reverse disease and promote longevity. Many of the nutrients found in these recommended food-based supplements and herbs are missing in our modern diets. By adding them back in, you have the opportunity to take both your keto diet and your health to the next level.

CHAPTER 6

Keto Lifestyle Tactics

How to Use Essential Oils, Stress Reduction, and Exercise

The word "diet" can be surprisingly misleading. It sounds like it's solely about food—change what you eat, and you're all good. But if you're focused only on what's on your plate, you're missing the bigger picture. Your lifestyle, your stress levels, even your thoughts can have a big impact on your health.

In Chapter 4, I encouraged you to start thinking like an Olympian when it comes to food choices. In this chapter, you'll see why it's important to extend that be-the-best-you-can-be mind-set to your lifestyle. That may sound like a tall order. But the strategies I recommend here are actually simple. They're small changes—using essential oils to support your body's healing and tweaking your daily habits to maximize your energy and bolster your mood—that will make a significant difference.

The following lifestyle hacks are based on ancient wisdom but have also been proven to be effective by leading-edge medical science—and they affect your health on the deepest level, transforming everything from the functioning of your cells to the activity of the genes that control things like aging and metabolic rate. They even change your brain, building up the centers where thinking and memory occur and minimizing those that promote fear and negative thinking. By utilizing these tactics and integrating them into your routine, you'll supercharge my keto diet program's effectiveness and set yourself up for a lifetime of good health.

THE NINE ESSENTIAL OILS THAT AMPLIFY HEALING

Essential oils have been used for more than three thousand years and are referenced in Egyptian, Greek, Ayurvedic, and Chinese medicine. They're also used in biblical medicine and are referenced more than two hundred times in the Bible.[1] These healing oils can be used to detoxify the body, bolster metabolism and brain function, and fight aging—intensifying the effects of the keto diet. High-quality essential oils can help you take your keto experience to the next level. Here are nine of my favorites, including how to utilize them to treat a variety of common conditions. In most cases, it's safe to apply an essential oil directly to your skin, but I've indicated the oils that should be diluted with a carrier oil, like coconut, jojoba, or olive oil. Use 5 drops of essential oil to 1 teaspoon of a carrier oil.

Clary sage is a flower from the clary sage plant. When it's distilled into an oil, the main chemical component is linalyl acetate, a substance that produces a sense of relaxation and is a powerful antioxidant. Clary sage can bolster the effects of the keto diet in a variety of other ways as well. It contains natural plant estrogens, so it can rejuvenate estrogen levels, support the long-term health of the uterus, and balance hormones, as well as ease menstrual cramps, heavy flow, and hot flashes. It's also a natural sedative, so it can relieve insomnia and stress—both of which contribute to inflammation.

How to use: To balance hormones, apply 3 drops several times a day to your abdomen (but don't use it during pregnancy, because it can cause contractions). To promote restfulness, apply 1 or 2 drops to your neck or the soles of your feet.

Fenugreek is an herb that blossoms during the summer and produces lovely white flowers. It can reduce inflammation and promote weight loss by improving the efficiency of insulin, enhancing keto's natural inflammation- and insulin-taming effects. Another important benefit: It can bolster testosterone. One study found that fenugreek supplements bolster men's sexual arousal, energy, and stamina and help maintain normal testosterone levels.[2]

How to use: Fenugreek can cause irritation when applied directly to the skin, so add 5 drops to 1 teaspoon of a carrier oil and massage it into the skin on your abdomen once or twice a day.

Frankincense comes from a small shrub with white or pale pink flowers and is often called the "king of oils" because it's so incredibly therapeutic. It can be beneficial for relieving chronic stress and anxiety, reducing pain and inflammation, boosting immunity, and even combating tumors—benefits that dovetail nicely with the keto diet's. A 2011 study found that frankincense oil has anti-inflammatory effects in the treatment of gingivitis and can reduce plaque and the depth of pockets around teeth.[3]

How to use: Diffuse it during prayer or meditation to promote peace and relaxation, or rub a few drops on your temples, your wrists, and the soles of your feet to promote internal healing.

Holy basil is an adaptogenic herb, which means it can help the body adapt to stress and exert a moderating effect on hormones, like thyroid hormones, that have become out of balance—all of which enhances the healing environment that the keto diet creates. It has a rich history as both a therapeutic and a sacred plant, with its use dating back more than three thousand years.

How to use: To support proper thyroid function, take 1 drop orally with 1 tablespoon of olive oil in a glass of water. To decrease stress and anxiety, inhale for a couple of minutes using a diffuser or rub a few drops on your temples.

Lavender's lovely purple blooms have been used for medicinal and religious purposes for more than twenty-five hundred years—and it's the most commonly used essential oil today because it has such a wide variety of uses. I recommend it to people on the keto diet for a couple of reasons. First, lavender is calming. A 2013 study found that taking 80 milligrams of lavender oil orally via capsules alleviated insomnia, anxiety, and depression,[4] and another study found that lavender oil reduces depression by nearly a third in people suffering from post-traumatic stress disorder.[5]

How to use: To promote sleep, apply 2 or 3 drops to the back of your neck, chest, and temples. To relieve anxiety and stress, add a few drops of lavender oil to a warm bath. To combat high blood pressure and soothe stress, diffuse lavender into the air throughout the day.

Lemon oil has been used to treat a wide spectrum of illnesses for a thousand years. Lemon essential oil has strong antistress effects. In a study of mice it had antidepressant-like effects, and lemon oil aromatherapy was found to reduce nausea and vomiting during pregnancy. In traditional Chinese medicine, lemon oil is used to combat conditions related to dampness, like colds, candida, diarrhea, respiratory infections, and sore throats. Lemon oil is great for supporting overall health during your keto diet.

How to use: To clear mucus and phlegm, inhale lemon oil directly from the bottle or mix 5 drops with 1 teaspoon of a carrier oil and apply it topically to your chest and nose. To ease seasonal allergies, take 1 or 2 drops orally, mixed with equal parts peppermint and lavender and a carrier oil. To improve mood, diffuse it in the air or apply a drop or two to your wrists and chest. Don't apply lemon oil to your skin before going out in the sun, because it can make you more sensitive to UV rays.

Peppermint was used in ancient Egyptian, Chinese, and Japanese folk medicine. It has a cooling, calming effect on the body and can help relieve sore muscles and headaches. It also soothes respiratory and digestive conditions—a 2007 study found that after four weeks patients with irritable bowel syndrome reported an average 50 percent reduction in symptoms.[6] Its effects are a nice complement to my keto program.

How to use: To relieve muscle pain, dilute 2 to 4 drops and apply it topically to the area in need of relief. For headaches, rub a drop or two on your forehead and temples. For digestive trouble, apply a dab to your abdomen, and for respiratory conditions diffuse it or add 10 drops to 2 cups of boiling water; pour the water into a heatproof bowl on the counter, drape a towel loosely over your head and the bowl (keeping your face well above the hot water), and breathe in the aroma for 5 minutes.

Rosemary is also a member of the mint family, and ancient cultures diffused it to disinfect the air and prevent sickness from spreading. It's now known for being able to support the healing of neurological tissue and boost brain function—one of the main benefits of the keto diet as well. A 2012 study found it improved subjects' cognitive performance and mood.[7] It can also help detoxify the body, improve hair growth, and help restore the body's hormonal balance.

How to use: For cognitive function, apply it topically to your nose and forehead. For detoxification, apply 2 to 3 drops to your abdomen. To promote hair growth, apply 3 to 5 drops to your scalp, rub it in, and allow it to sit for 5 minutes before rinsing. For better hormonal balance and reduced inflammation, add 1 to 2 drops to a glass of water and drink it.

Tea tree oil is made from the leaves of the plant *Melaleuca alternifolia* and has been used for thousands of years by the Aborigines of Australia. The oil has antiseptic properties and can be helpful for treating wounds because it can kill a variety of bacteria, viruses, and fungi. A 2007 study found it can also be effective for treating acne,[8] and it's often used for other skin conditions such as dandruff, psoriasis, eczema, toenail fungus, and ringworm. It's a good oil to have in your treatment arsenal.

How to use: To clean and disinfect cuts, combine 2 drops of tea tree oil with 2 drops of lavender oil and apply to the area. To treat acne, create a face wash by mixing 5 drops of tea tree oil with 2 tablespoons of raw honey. For dandruff, add 5 drops of tea tree oil to shampoo or conditioner. For psoriasis or eczema, make a soothing lotion by combining 5 drops of tea tree oil, 5 drops of lavender oil, and 1 teaspoon of coconut oil; apply it topically twice a day. For toenail fungus and ringworm, apply a few drops topically to the affected area.

TACKLING STRESS: THE PLAGUE OF MODERN LIFE

Think about how often you run into friends or acquaintances on the street, and in response to the usual "How are you?" they say one word: "Busy." It almost feels like a badge of honor to say how crazy our lives have become. And yet, we all know how much better off we'd be, physically and mentally, if we could only get stress under control and find forms of relief that really work. While stress can be a positive, motivating factor when you're under pressure to perform well at work, to ace an important exam, or to achieve a personal best in an athletic competition, more and more research shows that *chronic stress*, the kind that settles in and makes us miserable day after day, is as dangerous for the body as poor diet, lack of sleep, or a sedentary lifestyle. Too much stress also promotes weight gain and can make it difficult to stick to my keto diet program.

As many as 75 percent of all visits to the doctor's office are for conditions caused by stress.[9] Here's why: When you feel you're under threat, the sympathetic, or activating, branch of your nervous system takes the helm. A tiny region at the base of your brain known as the hypothalamus sets off an alarm, preparing your body to fight or flee. Your adrenal glands, located on top of each kidney, release adrenaline, which increases your heart rate, elevates your blood pressure, and sends energy to your muscles, as well as cortisol, which floods your bloodstream with glucose and tamps down your immune responses, digestive system, and reproductive systems—anything that's not essential for the physical challenge your body thinks it's facing. When stress doesn't go away, your system is awash in cortisol 24/7, causing inflammation and creating wear and tear on every cell in your body. Over time, exposure to high levels of cortisol increases your risk for heart disease, diabetes, weight gain or obesity, depression, anxiety, sleep problems, cognitive impairment, autoimmune diseases, digestive disorders, and even cancer.

Toxic? You bet. And completely counterproductive for achieving your keto goals. When you're stressed, it's easier to reach for comforting carbs than stick with your keto plan.

That's why it's incumbent on each and every one of you to find ways to soothe your nervous system and teach your body how to calm down. Activities that engage the parasympathetic branch of the nervous system (PNS), also known as the "rest and digest" system, help you recover from fight-or-flight mode. The PNS lowers cortisol, reduces blood pressure, and directs blood back to your digestive, reproductive, and immune systems. It calms the mind and soothes the heart and reverses chronic inflammation.

The sympathetic and parasympathetic nervous systems should act like the scales of justice, tilting one way in one situation, the other way in another, but ultimately balancing out. In our culture and our lives, there are too many factors weighing down the sympathetic side of the scale. So we need to consciously adopt lifestyle habits that tip the scales the other way. It's important for our peace of mind, our relationships, and our health. Here are seven of the best ways to restore balance to your nervous system, create an internal environment that promotes healing, and infuse your everyday life with powerful moments of calm so you can get the most out of your keto journey.

Take healing baths with lavender oil and Epsom salts before bed. A detoxifying bath is one of the best ways to put your body into a parasympathetic state before going to sleep. Add 20 drops of lavender oil and 1 cup of Epsom salts, which is high in magnesium, a mineral that promotes relaxation, to a hot bath and soak for 20 minutes. Your temperature naturally drops as you sleep. By raising your body's internal temperature a degree or two before bed, you'll experience a steeper drop during the night, which may help you sleep more deeply.

Pray and meditate for 10 minutes a day. Contemplative practices like prayer, meditation, and visualization can quiet the jumble of stress-producing thoughts crowding your mind—creating a sense of ease that can carry throughout the day. Practiced regularly, calming the mind can help you approach life's ups and downs with greater equanimity. It also can reduce blood pressure, anxiety, and pain and may help with insomnia. Meditation has been widely studied over the past twenty years, and research shows that it actually sculpts the brain in healthy ways, decreasing the strength of both the "default mode network,"[10] the brain region that is active when we're ruminating and worrying, and the amygdala, the brain's fear center.[11] While it turns down the volume on worry and fear, meditation also increases connectivity in brain regions responsible for emotion regulation, learning, and memory,[12] helping you stay more composed as you move through your day. There are plenty of guided forms of these activities in app form or online, or you can easily do them on your own.

Practice gratitude. This simple habit can have profound benefits. I take a few minutes every day to take stock of all the good things in my life and thank God for all of his favor and grace. These moments of consciously focusing on my blessings help me put my stressors in perspective and balance the negative thoughts that can increase tension and decrease happiness. Thinking about things we appreciate triggers the parasympathetic branch of the nervous system, and studies show it can reduce blood pressure, improve immune function, and optimize sleep. One research paper in the *Journal of Health Psychology* found that a two-week gratitude intervention lowered women's blood pressure,[13] and another study by researchers at the University of California San Diego School of Medicine found that people with asymptomatic heart failure who were more grateful actually had lower inflammation.[14] One easy way to make this healing habit part of your routine: Every night before bed, write down five things you're grateful for. They don't have to be big things and they don't have to be things that are happening in your life at the moment. Think of things in the past you're grateful for as well. For instance, you can make note of anything from the friendly checker at the grocery store to a loved one's successful recovery from surgery last year. But be specific. Here's an example of what I might say: "God, I'm grateful for my loving wife and someone I can laugh with like we did with the kids this morning at breakfast." Focus on people, rather than things, since social connections provide more meaning in the long run.

Get social. Dozens of studies have shown that people who have satisfying relationships with family and friends and their larger communities are happier, have fewer health problems, and live longer.[15] Supportive interactions with others bolster immune, cardiovascular, and hormonal function and reduce "allostatic load"—the wear and tear on the body created by stress.

Engage with nature. Most of us spend so much time hunched in front of our computers we forget there's a big, beautiful world outside—but there's so much to gain if we can carve out time for a walk in the woods, a picnic in the park, or a trip to the beach. A study in *Environmental Health and Preventive Medicine* found that people who strolled through a forest had lower blood pressure and levels of cortisol afterward than those who walked around a city.[16] Even better, being in nature can inspire feelings of awe, wonder, gratitude, and reverence—

positive emotions that not only lead to increased well-being and physical health but also can motivate us to be more generous, cooperative, and kind (and doing good for others can reduce stress as well). In other words, a quiet stroll in the park can trigger a cascade of stress-reducing emotions that leave us better off in numerous ways.

Get at least eight hours of sleep. Forty percent of people in the United States get fewer than seven hours of sleep a night, and the average amount of shut-eye is 6.8 hours—more than an hour less than people got in 1942.[17] It doesn't seem like a big deal to skimp on sleep—especially when your life is busy and there are so many items on your to-do list. But those hours you spend in bed make a great deal of difference to your health, because that's when most of the deep, restorative healing takes place inside your cells. In fact, sleep deprivation has been linked to high blood pressure, heart disease, diabetes, and weight gain. In other words, lack of sleep can sabotage your efforts to get healthy on the keto diet. Take weight loss. When you stay up binge-watching or surfing the web and shortchange your sleep, the level of the hunger hormone, ghrelin, increases by as much as 15 percent, according to a study in *PLOS Medicine*. While ghrelin makes you hungrier, daytime fatigue undermines your ability to resist eating—a double whammy that leads to weight gain. Indeed, the *PLOS Medicine* study, which included more than a thousand people, found that in those who slept fewer than eight hours a night, body mass index increased in proportion to lost sleep.[18]

Rethink your schedule. It's supereasy to say yes to every project and event that comes your way—and literally schedule yourself into stress. If you're guilty of this (I know I am), it can help to take a few minutes to think about your priorities. Identify the three to five things that mean the most to you and structure your life so they receive the bulk of your time and energy. In order to do that, you need to learn to say no. It's a challenge for most of us. But it can help to learn to say no gracefully. Thank people for the opportunity, express admiration for their efforts, but explain assertively that it's just not going to work for you this time. To stay strong, remind yourself that if you say yes you'll be spending time on someone else's priorities, not your own.

Place limits on technology. Fully 20 percent of people say they "constantly" monitor their social media feeds, and most check their phones within fifteen minutes of waking up.[19] But the onslaught of information can make you feel overwhelmed, triggering the fight-or-flight response. To keep it in check, take tech breaks every few hours. Go for a walk without your phone; get up from your computer and chat with a friend. Shut off all your devices a couple of hours before bedtime (the blue light can interfere with sleep), and try to stay away from technology as much as you can on weekends.

WHY EXERCISE IS A STAPLE OF THE KETO DIET

If you exercise regularly already, congratulations! I encourage you to keep it up. If you don't, it's time to start. Exercise is a critical component of my keto diet program because it works synergistically with the diet to restore your health and help you shed weight. Whether you do a gentle yoga class, lift weights, or take a 3-mile run, exercise offers a host of remarkable benefits. Strength training and cardiovascular exercise are both important, and I recommend doing a mix of the two to keep your muscles strong and your heart healthy. The amount of time you spend can vary. If you're doing strenuous exercise, like interval training, in which you alternate 30-second sprints with 90 seconds of walking or jogging—a great way to increase the fat loss of the keto diet—you can get away with 15 minutes a day. If you're walking or doing yoga, aim for 45 to 60 minutes of exercise almost every day, even if it doesn't all happen in one session.

The payoffs begin with stress reduction. During exercise, your body releases gamma-aminobutyric acid, or GABA, a calming neurotransmitter. A mere 20-minute workout can improve your mood for up to 12 hours,[20] partly because it also prompts a rise in three other substances: brain-derived neurotrophic factor, which can repair damage in the brain caused by stress and depression; endorphins, your brain's feel-good chemicals; and endocannabinoids, your body's natural cannabis-like compound, which promotes relaxation and well-being.

While you're sweating, you're also remodeling your body to make it more resistant to disease. A German review of fifteen long-term exercise studies found that regular physical activity not only helps control weight but also reduces the risk of heart disease, type 2 diabetes, and dementia, including Alzheimer's.[21] Not surprisingly, exercise has also been shown to help you live longer. When researchers from Harvard University, the National Cancer Institute, and other institutions pooled data on people's workout habits from six large health surveys, they found that the greatest longevity boost came from exercising at a moderate intensity 450 minutes a week.[22] Compared to people who never exercised, those who worked out a little more than an hour a day were 39 percent less likely to die prematurely. Think about that. Just 1 hour a day is enough to transform your health—especially when you exercise in conjunction with a healthy keto diet.

TOP TIPS FOR EXERCISING ON A KETOGENIC DIET

Follow these tips to help boost weight loss and avoid side effects while on a ketogenic diet:

REDUCE YOUR EXERCISE LOAD TEMPORARILY

Keep workouts to a minimum for the first few days, until your body becomes more adjusted to being in ketosis.

Suggested workouts for the first few days include:

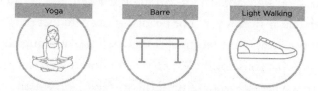

Yoga | Barre | Light Walking

REPLACE LONG BOUTS OF CARDIO WITH HIGH-INTENSITY INTERVAL TRAINING

1 Involves short bursts of high-intensity exercise followed by recovery periods

2 Lowers the bar of entry for exercisers

3 Takes less time to complete a workout

4 Burns fat faster

5 Helps build muscle mass

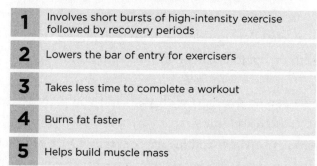

Find something you love to do so you'll stick with it. Yoga, barre, walking, jogging, swimming, cycling—they're all great options. I'm a fan of high-intensity interval training, in which you alternate between short bursts of high-intensity exercise and longer periods of low-intensity effort, because you can get in a great workout in 20 minutes—and research has shown it's a great way to burn fat.

To solidify your commitment, have regular exercise dates with friends. Maintaining social connections is a vital part of staying healthy, too; by combining these two powerhouse stay-well strategies, you maximize your time, your enjoyment, and your well-being.

And don't relegate exercise to an activity you do only in the gym or when you lace up your sneakers. Embrace movement every opportunity you get. Take a walk at lunchtime or after dinner. Stretch while you're watching TV. Do a few push-ups or jumping jacks to boost your energy when you're flagging at work. Movement floods our bodies with happiness-bolstering chemicals and makes us feel vital and alive. As the saying goes, "Good things come to those who sweat."

EATING OUT AND TRAVELING ON KETO

Here's a question I get asked a lot: If I'm on the keto diet, can I still go to restaurants? The answer is yes. The beauty of my keto diet program is that you can almost always find decent options when you're eating out. You just need to approach it consciously. When you're choosing a restaurant, opt for one that serves wholesome, organic, farm-to-table fare, where you're more likely to find entrées that dovetail with the diet. If you're meeting friends or colleagues somewhere less healthy, here are some general guidelines:

- For breakfast, have an omelet with goat cheese and vegetables.
- For dinner, opt for steak or salmon with a double order of sautéed vegetables.
- Bring a cut-up avocado with you, and you'll always have some healthy fat to add to your meal.
- Stay away from beer and sugary cocktails. Once or twice a week, you can have one or two glasses of sugar-free, dry-farmed organic wine

DINING OUT ON THE KETO DIET

Instead of ordering this...   Order this!

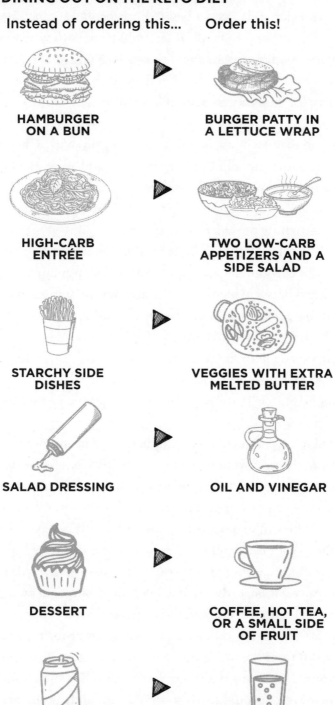

HAMBURGER ON A BUN → **BURGER PATTY IN A LETTUCE WRAP**

HIGH-CARB ENTRÉE → **TWO LOW-CARB APPETIZERS AND A SIDE SALAD**

STARCHY SIDE DISHES → **VEGGIES WITH EXTRA MELTED BUTTER**

SALAD DRESSING → **OIL AND VINEGAR**

DESSERT → **COFFEE, HOT TEA, OR A SMALL SIDE OF FRUIT**

SODA → **SPARKLING WATER**

or liquor with club soda, but it's best to limit alcohol as much as possible. Alcohol is dehydrating and pulls B vitamins from your system, so drink extra water — two glasses for every one glass of wine or cocktail — and supplement with a B-complex vitamin and milk thistle, a cleansing herb known for its ability to detoxify the liver.

Traveling may seem challenging, too, but my wife, Chelsea, and I follow these same guidelines for restaurants and pack plenty of keto snacks. Here are some of our favorites:

- Keto-friendly protein or collagen bars
- Grass-fed beef, wild-caught salmon, or organic chicken jerky that doesn't contain any unpronounceable ingredients
- Roasted nuts and seeds, like macadamia and pumpkin seeds
- Portable packets of almond or cashew butter
- Kale chips or seaweed chips
- Homemade keto granola, packed with nuts, shredded coconut, and cacao nibs (see Granola recipe on page 283), or my favorite almond butter–based Keto Fat Bombs (see recipe on page 279).

It's hard to be perfect, but do your best. And keep this in mind: On my program, the strict keto diet lasts only thirty days. Some of you may want to continue it for sixty or ninety days, max, if you have more weight to lose or stubborn health problems. But it's such a powerful approach and its effects kick in so quickly that you don't need to stay on strict keto forever. Once your thirty (or sixty or ninety) days are over and you're in the Forever Keto Cycling phase, you'll have two or three days a week when you can eat more carbs, so schedule your dinners out on those days. For more info on how to eat on those days, see Chapter 16.

Keto isn't just about losing weight. It's about restoring your body's natural health from the inside out. And in order to do that you need to expand your focus from the foods you're eating to the choices you're making in the rest of your life. By soothing your body with essential oils, taming stress, getting enough sleep, and exercising regularly, you'll heal your body, feel your best, and amplify the keto diet's therapeutic effects.

PART II

How the Keto Diet Heals Disease

CHAPTER 7

Keto Metabolism Makeover

How Healthy Fats Can Help You Lose Weight and Beat Diabetes

I was teaching an advanced nutrition workshop about how to use food as medicine when I met Kirby and Helen, a couple in their late fifties. She was a retired high school teacher and he was a college professor on the verge of retirement too. After the lecture, they introduced themselves, explained that they were interested in improving their health, and made an appointment for a consultation in my office.

During our consultation, I learned that Kirby, who was about fifty pounds overweight, had been diagnosed with type 2 diabetes and high cholesterol and was taking three medications—one to get his cholesterol under control and two for diabetes. Even so, he was struggling with back and leg pain, common neurological symptoms of the disease. Helen had about thirty pounds to lose and had been diagnosed with prediabetes. Her blood glucose levels were just below the cutoff for the full-blown disease.

I explained to them that the ketogenic diet is ideal for people with diabetes, an illness that's characterized by insulin resistance, in which cells no longer allow insulin, which carries the glucose cells use for fuel, inside. The result is high blood sugar and high insulin, a dangerous combination that leads to weight gain and a host of other health problems associated with diabetes.

But feeding the body healthy fat and virtually eliminating carbs is one of the quickest and most effective ways to get your insulin, blood sugar, and weight under control. Since carbohydrates are the foods that turn into glucose in your blood, when you stop eating them your blood sugar and insulin automatically plummet. As glucose and insulin decline, the body's cells have a chance to rest and recover, and, over time, their ability to respond normally to insulin is restored.

I gave Kirby and Helen a keto shopping list, along with recipes, including one for a daily smoothie made with avocado, coconut milk, keto-friendly protein powder, and two teaspoons of cinnamon, a spice that has been shown in some studies to lower blood sugar and cholesterol. I also recommended that they take chromium, a mineral that is necessary in small quantities for human health—and that can help control blood sugar in people with diabetes.

When I saw them two weeks later, Helen's blood sugar had already dropped back into the normal range, according to the A1c, the blood test that is used to diagnose the illness. She no longer had prediabetes. Two weeks after that, Kirby's A1c had dropped to 5.5 percent. Anything below 5.7 percent is considered normal, so he was able to safely go off his medications. His diabetes was reversed, too.

Within a few months, they'd both lost all the extra weight they'd built up during the years when their bodies were becoming increasingly resistant to insulin. They looked lean and healthy, and their energy returned. Every time I did a local lecture, they showed up, bright-eyed, enthusiastic, and engaged. I continued seeing them as patients until I stopped my full-time practice four years later. Throughout that time they remained committed to a keto lifestyle, their weight and blood sugar continued to be normal, and their overall health was vibrant.

Kirby and Helen's success with the ketogenic diet isn't unusual. A *European Journal of Clinical Nutrition* review of the medical literature assessing the diet's effectiveness for treating various health conditions concluded that the scientific evidence showing the approach can help with diabetes, weight loss, and cardiovascular disease is strong—as strong as the evidence for treating epilepsy,[1] a condition for which many neurologists today recommend keto. The studies' results are so convincing that the renowned Duke Lifestyle Medicine Clinic at Duke University School of Medicine uses the ketogenic diet as a first-line therapy for type 2 diabetes and obesity, and Virta Health, a telemedicine type 2 diabetes clinic, counsels patients on using it to reverse their disease.[2]

Diabetes and obesity limit your ability to stay active and vital with age, cause untold suffering, contribute to heart disease, and cut short far too many people's lives. By eating wholesome, nutrient-dense fat for fuel and virtually eliminating carbs, you remove most of the glucose from your blood and bring insulin back into a safe, nontoxic range, purging your body of the culprits behind these pervasive illnesses that plague the modern world. Here's a look at the science of why and how the ketogenic diet can turn the tide.

WHY THE KETO DIET IS SO EFFECTIVE FOR WEIGHT LOSS

A number of years ago, a former offensive lineman in the NFL came to me because he wanted to lose weight. He was a big guy when he was playing—he needed to be for his career—but in the years since he had retired he had gained more weight. When I met him, he was forty-one and carrying an extra 165 pounds. He'd never heard of the ketogenic diet, but when I told him why a healthy-fat, low-carb approach was the most effective way to shed pounds, he instinctively got it—and agreed to give it a try.

Over the next couple of months, he began losing weight quickly. His wife, who was about seventy pounds overweight, was so impressed she began the keto diet as well. Within several months they had both reached a healthy weight—and he looked like the fit athlete he had been in his prime. Three years later, I was at a mall in Nashville when I ran into his wife. She told me they had eventually shifted to keto cycling, and they'd been adhering to that approach, with intermittent full-keto bouts thrown in, for years. She looked fit, trim, and vibrant. I was impressed with their commitment—and reminded of the power of keto to help people regain not only their health but also their sense of themselves. Excess weight can make you feel like you're living in a stranger's body — and the football player's wife said as much to me that day in the mall. When we parted, she hugged me and thanked me for changing their lives.

Although much of the weight-loss industry and medical field continues to adhere to the concept that shedding pounds is strictly about consuming fewer calories than you expend, anyone who has been paying attention to the medical literature for the past decade knows that's not accurate. A number of studies have shown that people who consume a low-carbohydrate diet lose more weight, especially during the first three to six months, than those eating more carbs and less fat — and a thorough review of the literature in the *British Journal of Nutrition* that looked at thirteen randomized controlled trials that lasted a year or more concurred: "Individuals assigned to a very-low-carbohydrate ketogenic diet achieved greater long-term reductions in body weight… than those assigned to a low fat diet," the researchers concluded.[3]

Keto is a successful weight-loss approach because it affects your body on a metabolic level, recalibrating its internal dials to healthier settings. It not only helps you lose weight quickly and naturally but also allows you to avoid many of the problems that come with traditional low-calorie diets.

As I explained in Chapter 1, ketosis affects your metabolism in remarkably positive ways. While most diets can help you lose weight, they also cause your metabolic rate to take a nosedive, so you burn fewer calories throughout the day. The ketogenic diet doesn't trigger this weight gain–promoting metabolic slowdown. In a study published in *Diabetes & Metabolic Syndrome: Clinical Research & Reviews*, researchers randomly assigned a group of thirty overweight adults with metabolic syndrome to one of three groups: a ketogenic diet with no exercise, a standard American diet with no exercise, or a standard American diet with three to five days a week of 30 minutes of exercise.[4] After ten weeks, the ketogenic group lost significantly more weight and body fat — and their metabolic rate was ten times higher than that of the two other groups. Similarly, in an eight-week randomized trial with twenty-six obese participants, those on a higher-fat diet lost 11 percent of their body fat while those on a standard, carbohydrate-based, low-fat diet lost just 2.1 percent.[5]

The secret to my keto diet's effectiveness can also be traced to its healthy influence on the following hormones underlying hunger, satiety, and weight gain:

Insulin. I've already explained how insulin promotes fat storage and weight gain. The keto diet is one of the most effective ways to turn around cells' insulin resistance (which leads to excess insulin in the blood) and interrupt this far-too-prevalent process. In one of the longest, most thorough real-world studies of the ketogenic diet and diabetes, published in *Diabetes Therapy* in 2018, researchers followed 218 diabetes patients on a low-carb, healthy-fat diet for a full year.[6] At the same time, they tracked 87 patients who received the usual diabetes care and a typical diet. Patients in the low-carb group were monitored to ensure that they remained in ketosis and advised to consume plenty of healthy omega-3, omega-6, monounsaturated, and saturated fats to bolster satiety and curb overeating. By the end of the year, the ketosis group had reduced their weight by 12 percent, on average. In addition, 72 percent of the ketosis group had an A1c less than 6.5 percent—meaning they no longer had full-blown diabetes and were either in the normal or prediabetes blood sugar range—and 94 percent of those who had been prescribed insulin reduced or discontinued their use. At the same time, their levels of HOMA-IR, a measure of insulin resistance, were reduced by 55 percent. Participants in the usual care group, by contrast, remained as sick as ever. They had no changes in weight, A1c levels, or medication use.

In a separate study in the journal *Lipids*, researchers put overweight people who had unhealthy blood lipid profiles (high triglycerides and LDL cholesterol and low HDL cholesterol) on either a carbohydrate-restricted diet or a low-fat diet for twelve weeks.[7] By the end of the study, fasting insulin had decreased nearly 50 percent in the low-carb group compared to just 19 percent in the low-fat group—and their decreases in abdominal fat showed similar disparities; the low-carb group lost 827 grams of fat while the low-fat group lost 506.

Gastrointestinal hormones involved in hunger and satiety. Research has repeatedly found that people on a keto diet don't get as hungry as those on traditional weight-loss diets. One reason is that the diet's high concentration of healthy fats, along with plentiful veggies, makes it extremely satisfying. There's no need to count calories, because you actually feel full naturally after eating less food. In addition, the keto diet seems to be the only weight-loss approach, aside from fasting, that has a positive effect on a number of key hormones that play a role in hunger and fullness. Many of these hormones originate in the gut, where they assess food qualities and quantities and send signals to the brain telling you to keep eating or stop. Ghrelin, for instance, is produced in the stomach and stimulates hunger. On a typical low-calorie weight-loss diet, ghrelin levels rise, increasing your urge to eat and making you crave high-calorie, high-carb foods. But the keto diet suppresses ghrelin—and does so for as long as you stay in ketosis, according to studies published in the *European Journal of Clinical Nutrition*[8] and *Frontiers in Psychology*.[9] At the same time, it maintains a healthy level of cholecystokinin (CCK), a peptide produced in the small intestine that causes you to reduce food intake, meal size, and duration. With a typical weight-loss diet, CCK and a variety of other peptides that play a role in reducing food intake experience a long-lasting decrease, making weight regain much more likely.

Leptin. The main job of leptin, a hormone produced by your body's fat cells, is to signal the hypothalamus, one part of the brain involved in hunger and satiety, that it's time to put the fork down. Obesity is often thought of as a problem of leptin resistance, when your brain is starving but your body is obese. Overeating can cause leptin resistance, and typical weight-loss diets cause the hormone to plummet, dulling your ability to intuit when you're full, according to a study in the *New England Journal of Medicine*.[10] Foods that are most likely to interfere with leptin levels are those high in added sugar, unhealthy fat like trans fats, artificial flavors and sweeteners, refined grains, and other synthetic ingredients—but healthy fats, high-fiber veggies, and healthy protein seem to counteract that effect and allow leptin to continue functioning normally.[11]

REVERSING DIABETES WITH THE KETO DIET

In Chapter 2, I explained a bit about how the ketogenic diet can help with diabetes—a disease that's wreaking havoc on our population. Nearly half of adults in the United States have diabetes or prediabetes.[12] As heartbreaking, the illness affects a growing number of children. Thirty years ago, type 2 diabetes was nearly unheard of in anyone under twenty.[13] But its incidence began to spike in the mid-1990s, and since 2002 the rate of new cases has grown nearly 5 percent every year, according to a recent study in the *New England Journal of Medicine*.[14] When diabetes starts early, its dangerous complications, like heart disease, stroke, kidney failure, vision loss, and limb loss, can occur at younger ages—meaning a growing population of children may end up suffering the devastating consequences of the illness by their forties or fifties, or earlier, unless we find ways to stop it.

That's where my keto diet program comes in. A growing trove of evidence shows that a diet high in healthy fats and very low in carbs is a safe, effective way to tackle this modern menace—including in children. In a study of fifty-eight obese children in the *Journal of Pediatric Endocrinology and Metabolism*, researchers placed half of the group on a carb-restricted diet and the other half on a regular low-calorie diet for six months.[15] By the end of the trial, both groups had lost significant amounts of weight and body fat and reduced their fasting insulin—but the declines were more pronounced in the ketogenic group.

But let's start from the beginning: What causes type 2 diabetes and insulin resistance in the first place? Studies point to sugar as the likely culprit—and most people consume way too much. The average American devours 19.5 teaspoons, or 82 grams, every day[16]—that's sixty-six pounds of added sugar a year!—an amount that soars far beyond even the generous American Heart Association recommendation of 6 teaspoons a day for women and 9 teaspoons for men. Considering that a single can of soda has 11 teaspoons of sugar, you can see how easy it is to overdo it on the sweet stuff.

Research in *PLOS One* that looked at diabetes rates and food intake in 175 countries found that every 150 calories of sugar (about the amount in one can of soda) per person per day was associated with an increased prevalence of the disease.[17] The effect was so pronounced that the researchers concluded that differences in sugar availability explain variations in diabetes prevalence in disparate populations, regardless of their rates of physical activity, overweight, or obesity. Diabetes is so closely linked to carbs and sugar that some researchers have started calling insulin resistance "carbohydrate intolerance."

When you consume too much added sugar, your blood glucose levels increase, prompting the pancreas to secrete more insulin. High levels of insulin direct the body to store calories as fat, leading to weight gain. Insulin also affects leptin, the hormone in the body that works as a natural appetite suppressant. When our bodies no longer respond to leptin signals telling us we're full, we overeat and gain weight. High glucose plus high insulin plus weight gain are the key ingredients of diabetes.

But even as evidence of the dangers of sugar has piled up, the medical community has been slow to adopt the ketogenic approach for diabetes, partly because of the lingering fear of dietary fat that exists in mainstream medicine. Now, finally, that outdated attitude may be gradually changing. In its most recent paper on diet for diabetes, the American Diabetes Association acknowledges that fat quality is more important than quantity[18]—and points out that a systematic review of the literature, as well as four individual studies and a meta-analysis published since the review, have found that lowering fat intake doesn't improve blood sugar control or cardiovascular disease risk factors.

Meanwhile, more and more studies are showing that a diet high in healthy fats and low in carbs and added sugars can turn diabetes around. In the prior section, I mentioned a yearlong study of the ketogenic diet in overweight diabetes patients, which found that 94 percent of those on a ketogenic diet were able to reduce or discontinue their use of insulin. The study also found that 42 percent of the keto dieters whose blood sugar had dropped below the diabetic zone were able to stop taking their diabetes medications. In other words, as their blood sugar levels normalized, their insulin did too, and their bodies were able to resume healthy functioning without medication. Their blood tests revealed other healthy changes as well, including reductions in markers of inflammation and triglycerides (fat in the blood), as well as improvements in liver function.

Similar findings came from a six-month study in *Experimental & Clinical Cardiology*.[19] Researchers followed eighty-three obese diabetes patients with high glucose and high cholesterol and found that their weight and BMI decreased significantly on a ketogenic diet (by the end they lost an average of thirty-two pounds)—and they also showed meaningful decreases in blood glucose levels, total cholesterol, LDL (bad) cholesterol, and triglycerides, while their HDL (good) cholesterol increased.

Even those remarkable results may not tell the whole story. The diets in these two long-term studies were healthy and put patients into ketosis, but they included a higher carbohydrate content and lower proportion of superhealthy fat than my keto diet program. In my practice, I learned that when you raise the bar by slashing carbs and loading up on the most nutritious types of fat, the positive effects on insulin, weight, blood sugar, cholesterol, and triglycerides can be even more dramatic. My keto diet plan contains no added sugar, which can help reduce your risk for diabetes as well as heart disease, fatty liver disease, and certain types of cancer, including colon and breast.

Studies of the ketogenic diet have found that it's safe for diabetics. But it's important to have your blood sugar monitored when you're using keto to manage diabetes, because your need for medication and insulin is likely to change quickly as your levels of blood glucose and insulin normalize.

THE NINE METABOLIC WONDER FOODS THAT MAKE YOU A CALORIE-BURNING MACHINE

The keto diet outstrips virtually every other eating program available when it comes to reversing diabetes and promoting weight loss. And you can maximize its healthful effects by supplementing the core diet with keto-friendly foods that bolster its natural metabolic benefits. Here are the nine options I always recommend to patients who have metabolic disease or want to lose weight. (For more metabolism-boosting advice to help you drop pounds fast, go to www.draxe.com/keto-diet -metabolism.)

Exogenous ketones can get you into ketosis more quickly and help you stay there — both of which can bolster weight loss and allow you to consistently and reliably reduce glucose and insulin, thereby reversing diabetes risk. If you have a powdered form, take 6 grams once or twice a day, with the first dose in the morning. If you have capsules, which are usually combined with synergistic ingredients, take 2 grams.

Bone broth protein powder promotes a feeling of fullness and contains glycine, an amino acid that's good for building muscle strength and controlling blood sugar. Add a scoop to your favorite keto-friendly beverage once or twice a day.

MCT (medium-chain triglycerides) oil is a type of fatty acid derived from coconut oil — and it's great for weight loss because it boosts fat burning. After you digest MCT oil, it's sent directly to your liver, where it has a thermogenic effect, making your metabolic engine run at a higher speed. In a study published in the *International Journal of Obesity and Related Metabolic Disorders*, participants who ate a diet rich in medium-chain triglycerides lost more body fat than those eating a diet high in long-chain fatty acids[20] — probably because the MCTs revved their metabolism and allowed them to burn more fat. Take 1 tablespoon in a smoothie or other beverage (you can take it straight, too) once to three times every day.

Chromium plays a role in the body's insulin-signaling pathway and can enhance the role of insulin. It also supports a healthy metabolism, since it can help you better absorb and distribute the nutrients you take in from your diet. A study conducted by the U.S. Department of Agriculture's Human Nutrition Research Center found that people with diabetes who were given a chromium supplement for four months had lower insulin and cholesterol than those given a placebo.[21] Other studies have found that people with higher intakes of chromium have less body fat and are better able to control their eating. For anyone with insulin resistance or diabetes, it's a good idea to take a multivitamin with 200 micrograms of chromium.

Warming seasonings that rev up your metabolism. You can take these in supplement form by following the dosage directions on the bottle or use liberally in your cooking:

- *Turmeric* can be helpful for managing diabetes. An animal study published in *Biochemical and Biophysical Research Communications* found that the curcumin in turmeric has a more potent effect on AMPK, an enzyme involved in lowering blood sugar, than metformin, a commonly prescribed diabetes drug.[22] It is also anti-inflammatory and can lower inflammatory markers associated with diabetes.

- *Ginger* has anti-inflammatory properties and can help regulate blood sugar as well. In one study, ginger supplementation actually reduced fasting blood sugar by 12 percent and improved long-term blood sugar control by 10 percent.[23]

- *Cinnamon* is good for the heart because it reduces cholesterol, triglycerides, and blood pressure—and it can help fight diabetes by lowering blood sugar levels and improving insulin sensitivity.

- *Cayenne pepper* has been found to reduce appetite. Those who consume it with their breakfast (I like to sprinkle it on my eggs) tend to eat fewer calories throughout the day. It also promotes fat burning and is a potent anti-inflammatory.

- *Peppercorns* are antioxidants that help stabilize blood sugar. Research published in the *Proceedings of the National Academy of Sciences* found that piperine, a substance in peppercorns, accelerates metabolism[24]—making it an effective tool for weight loss and diabetes control.

As the years tick by, our nation and our world continue to get sicker and fatter—and the more pills and diet programs doctors prescribe, the worse the problem becomes. But the ketogenic diet's unique ability to help you burn deep stores of dangerous body fat, boost metabolism, fight hunger, and transform high blood sugar and insulin offers a way forward. Whether you have five or fifty pounds to lose, my keto diet program can help you achieve your goals—and offers hope for a healthier tomorrow.

CHAPTER 8

Your Brain on Keto

How Ketosis Boosts Cognitive Performance and Protects Your Brain

In my second year of practice as a functional medicine doctor, I did a consultation with a new patient, Cheryl. She was thirty-four and had been diagnosed with multiple sclerosis (MS), a slow-progressing autoimmune inflammatory disease that affects the brain and spinal cord, causing back and extremity pain, weakness, fatigue, and muscle spasms. Most doctors believe there is no cure, and it tends to get worse over time, so the goal of treatment is to modify the course of the disease, slow its progression, and manage symptoms. By the time I met Cheryl, a wife and mother with two young children, she was so disabled she was in a wheelchair.

I suggested she try the ketogenic diet. It was a radical switch for her, because she was used to eating lots of carbs—and she and her husband, John, were skeptical that dietary changes alone could possibly make a difference. But I explained that the ketogenic diet is fundamentally different from any other approach to eating and walked them through the basics of how ketosis works. I told them that my nutritious high-fat, very-low-carb plan would stimulate her body to metabolize fat instead of glucose for fuel, and in doing so would significantly reduce the inflammation in her body and offer relief from her symptoms. They agreed to give it a try.

What happened next went beyond what most doctors think is possible. A couple of weeks later, when Cheryl came in for her next appointment, she was out of her wheelchair and using a walker. She said she was in less pain and had more energy. Two weeks after that she was walking on her own. By the time I saw her three months after her initial consultation, her MS symptoms had disappeared. John told me he felt like he had his wife back. Cheryl, a former athlete, had exercised for the first time in years. They were both in tears. We all hugged. It was a moment I won't forget.

Not long before I met Cheryl, I read a paper by a team of researchers from the National Institutes of Health, Johns Hopkins Hospital, and the University of California, Davis.[1] They summarized the evidence from a number of studies showing that the ketogenic diet could have protective effects on a broad range of neurodegenerative disorders, like Alzheimer's disease and Parkinson's. MS is one such illness. So are amyotrophic lateral sclerosis (ALS, or Lou Gehrig's disease), and Huntington's disease. The research team also presented details from studies showing that the diet might be beneficial for other brain-based conditions, like autism, traumatic brain injury, and stroke.

Since the 1920s, when doctors first discovered that the ketogenic diet could reduce seizures in children with untreatable epilepsy, the medical community has recognized its power to relieve neurological disorders. Now, a growing body of research is shedding light on how and why putting the body into a state of ketosis is able to improve the symptoms of some conditions when nothing else can. I'll explain those fascinating findings in the coming pages. But the truth is, the keto diet is nourishing for *all* brains. It gives you what I call a "keto-brain." When the brain starts using ketone bodies for fuel, many people notice they can function at a higher cognitive level. Whether you're a student trying to learn and remember new information, a parent caring for your family, or a professional with a demanding career, you need the gray matter inside your skull to function its best. My keto diet program is a proven way to stay sharp, fend off age-related cognitive decline, and help prevent neurodegenerative disorders from gaining a foothold in the first place.

A POWERFUL NEW WEAPON IN THE FIGHT AGAINST BRAIN DISORDERS

Diseases that cause brain degeneration affect millions of people around the world—and the numbers are growing. Alzheimer's alone, the most common of these illnesses, takes an astronomical toll. There are an estimated 5.7 million people in the United States,[2] including one in ten people age sixty-five or older, who suffer from this common form of dementia—and the number is expected to jump to nearly 14 million by 2020, according to the Alzheimer's Association.[3] Worldwide, 50 million people suffer from dementia, including Alzheimer's.[4] Add other neurodegenerative diseases like Parkinson's and MS, and you begin to see the scope of the problem. To make matters worse, there are few effective treatments for these devastating neurological disorders, and they often come with hefty price tags and problematic side effects. As a result, the ketogenic diet—an affordable option that can be beneficial for the brain as well as every other system in your body—has the potential to be a blessing for hundreds of millions of people.

Disorders that affect the brain and spinal cord respond well to the ketogenic approach because the brain runs more efficiently on ketones than on glucose, the sugary stuff that surges through your blood when you eat carbs. That's the fundamental reason you get keto-brain—a level of cognitive processing that makes you feel like you're cooking on all four burners. But the diet's effects go deeper. Studies show that it actually tweaks the body on a molecular level in ways that bolster neurological functioning.

Here's what cutting-edge science has revealed about the specific ways ketosis can protect you.

Alzheimer's

Every bite of food you put in your mouth fuels both your body and your brain—and your brain is *hungry*. It consumes an astounding 20 percent of your daily energy. But most of us have been feeding our brains the wrong stuff. Alarming new research shows that glucose, the fuel every carb eater's brain runs on, can damage this precious organ. A ten-year study of more than fifty-one hundred healthy people found that those with high blood sugar had faster rates of cognitive decline than those with normal blood sugar[5]—and the decline happened even in people whose blood sugar wasn't high enough to meet the clinical diagnosis of diabetes.

High glucose can be particularly dangerous for people who already have dementia. A study supported by the National Institute on Aging found a connection between higher glucose levels in the brains of Alzheimer's patients and the severity of their symptoms as well as the number of amyloid plaques and tangles, the disease's hallmark fingerprints.[6]

Given that, it's no surprise that research is starting to show that a ketogenic diet, which feeds the brain ketones instead of glucose, can support and protect your cognitive health. A study in mice with Alzheimer's found that those that were fed a ketogenic diet for forty-three days had a 25 percent decrease in the level of amyloid plaques in their brains.[7] And in the first human study, researchers at the University of Kansas put patients with mild Alzheimer's on a classic keto diet, including high doses of MCT oil supplements. After three months, participants' scores on a standard test of memory, language, and attention improved, on average, more than 5 points—a better result than achieved by any available Alzheimer's medication.[8] When the researchers tested the participants again four months after they went off the diet, their scores had dropped back to where they'd been at the study's outset—confirmation that the diet was responsible for participants' remarkable improvement.

Fueling your brain with ketones instead of glucose may help prevent Alzheimer's, too. One large study found that people with the lowest dietary carbohydrate intake were 80 percent less likely than those who ate the most carbs to develop mild cognitive impairment, a stepping-stone on the way to full-blown dementia.[9]

Again, the explanation lies, in part, in the ketogenic diet's ability to snuff out inflammation. There's evidence that reducing inflammation can be protective against age-related cognitive decline. For instance, one study found that people who took nonsteroidal anti-inflammatory medications like ibuprofen and naproxen for two or more years had a 40 percent reduced risk of this memory-stealing scourge.[10]

Oxidative damage from free radicals plays a role in the development of dementia as well—and the ketogenic diet is one of the most effective ways to turn on your body's innate protective mechanisms against damaging rogue molecules. Your cells have the ability to create antioxidant enzymes—similar to the ones you consume in antioxidant-rich foods like blueberries but far more potent. The system is activated by a protein in the cell's nucleus called Nrf2—and studies show that both consumption of omega-3 essential fatty acids and the ketogenic diet itself can trigger Nrf2 to swing into action. Ketosis flips the switch that brings your body's internal damage-control forces to life.

Multiple sclerosis

Most trials of the ketogenic diet for MS have been done in animals, but a study in Germany revealed that the positive results my patient Cheryl achieved may be typical. In a six-month randomized, controlled trial with patients who had been diagnosed with MS, German researchers divided participants into three groups: One continued eating their usual diet, a second fasted for seven days before returning to their usual diet, and a third consumed a ketogenic diet for the study's duration.[11] Participants in both the fasting group and the ketogenic group showed substantial improvement in symptoms. Everything from their energy levels and physical functioning to their cognitive ability and emotional well-being was better. The fasting group's benefits peaked at three months. But here's the really cool thing: The keto diet participants continued making steady, significant improvement over the six months of the study. Both the ketogenic diet and prolonged fasting relieved MS patients' symptoms, because they both put the body into ketosis. But the ketogenic diet provided the greatest degree of improvement.

Studies have uncovered two important reasons why eating a high-fat, very-low-carb diet can improve the symptoms of MS. First, inflammation plays a key role in the disease—just as it does with every other neurodegenerative disorder—and there's good evidence that the high fatty acid load of the ketogenic diet can activate the body's anti-inflammatory mechanisms. For example, studies show that fatty acids stimulate peroxisome proliferator-activated receptor alpha (PPARa), a protein that regulates the expression of certain genes and produces a potent anti-inflammatory response.[12]

Second, neurodegeneration occurs partly because the cells' mitochondria, or "energy factories," malfunction and fail to produce enough energy to meet the body's needs. The ketogenic diet has a number of favorable effects on mitochondria function.[13] It turns on genes that lead to mitochondrial replication, so you grow more of the structures that provide your body with energy; it lowers levels of damaging reactive oxygen species, so it protects those delicate, life-sustaining mitochondria within each cell; and it increases the availability of adenosine triphosphate (ATP), the vital molecules within mitochondria that function like a food delivery service, capturing chemical energy from the breakdown of food and shuttling it to the places within the cell where energy-consuming activities are taking place.

Parkinson's disease

The ability of the ketogenic diet to stimulate ATP production is critical in Parkinson's because the disease stems in large part from a defect in energy production at the level of the mitochondria. Studies in mice show that the administration of exogenous ketones from supplements improves the symptoms of the disease. And the only study that's been done in humans so far echoed those results. Researchers at Beth Israel Medical Center and St. Luke's Roosevelt Hospital Center in New York put Parkinson's patients on a ketogenic diet for twenty-eight days and found a 46 percent reduction, on average, in their scores on the Unified Parkinson's Disease Rating Scale[14]—a scale that measures patients' physical, cognitive, and emotional functioning as well as their ability to perform activities of daily living, like dressing themselves, feeding themselves, and going to the grocery store. One patient's scores improved 81 percent.

Autism

Autism has neurological roots, and like the neurodegenerative conditions we've been talking about, it is also associated with mitochondrial
dysfunction. Indeed, a number of studies in mice have shown that a
ketogenic diet can improve the symptoms of autism—and the case
reports and small studies that have been done in children show promise
as well. In one, forty-five children with autism were divided into three
groups and put on three separate diets—the ketogenic diet, a gluten-
free, casein-free (GFCF) diet that has shown potential in improving
symptoms in autistic children, and a typical balanced diet.[15] When the
researchers assessed the children after six months on each approach,
they found that those on both the keto and GFCF diets showed behavioral improvements and symptom reduction, but those on the keto diet
scored the highest on cognition and sociability—two core challenges
for children with autism.

Depression and anxiety

In controlled studies in animals, the keto diet and the administration of
exogenous ketones have both been found to reduce anxiety and depression in much the same way medication would.[16] In other words, keto-
brain boosts mood, too. The approach has yet to be thoroughly studied
in humans, but anecdotal reports of its effectiveness are ubiquitous—
and there are valid biological explanations for why ketosis might
enhance emotional well-being. For one thing, inflammation contributes to depression, and ketosis tames inflammation. At the same time,
the keto diet may increase GABA, an inhibitory neurotransmitter that
helps you feel calm. And burning ketones instead of glucose for fuel
prevents the spikes and dips of energy and mood that come with carb
consumption. Anyone who eats a high-carb diet knows the feeling of
being "hangry." That's what happens when you're burning glucose.
Blood sugar surges, then plummets. And when it drops, it affects your
mood. In addition to depression and anxiety, there's accruing evidence
that the keto diet can be helpful in other mental health issues as well,

including schizophrenia, bipolar disorder, and attention deficit hyper-activity disorder.

Headaches

The keto diet's ability to curb brain inflammation and enhance mito-chondria function could also explain recent findings that the diet is helpful for people with headache disorders. In a study reported in the *European Journal of Neurology*, researchers put forty-five migraine suffer-ers on a ketogenic diet for six months and compared them to fifty-one migraineurs following a standard low-calorie diet.[17] The number of attacks, number of days with headaches, and amount of medication participants needed dropped significantly in those following the keto-genic approach. In another hopeful study of people with drug-resistant cluster headaches (a series of short but extremely painful headaches), eleven of eighteen patients had full resolution of their condition and four had a 50 percent or more reduction in the number of attacks.[18]

HEALING YOUR GUT AFFECTS THE HEALTH OF YOUR BRAIN

You've probably made the comment "I have a gut feeling about this." The idea that your gut and brain are linked couldn't be more apt. The way you feel emotionally and the way your brain functions are inti-mately connected with your belly. For years, medicine viewed each part of the body in isolation. But the reality is, it's one, big, intercon-nected whole — like a symphony, where every player contributes to the overall functioning. And certain parts of the body have such a tight symbiosis that when something goes wrong with one, it nearly always affects the other. That's true of the gut and brain.

The gut is home to the enteric nervous system (ENS), made up of two thin layers of more than 500 million nerve cells — even more than the spinal cord. These cells line the gastrointestinal tract, from the esophagus to the stomach, small intestine, and colon, and manage every aspect of digestion by controlling blood flow, muscle contractions, and the secretion of gastric digestive juices. To do so, the ENS uses the same tools as your brain does: a complex network of neurons, neurotransmitters like serotonin and dopamine, and proteins. The ENS is known as the "second brain" because its structure and neurochemistry are essentially the same as what's inside your skull.[19] The two brains speak a similar neurochemical language, and they communicate constantly. As a result, when something goes wrong with the gut it can affect the brain, and vice versa.

Gastrointestinal symptoms are three to four times more common in children with autism than in typically developing children.[20] Patients with Parkinson's and Alzheimer's often have gut issues as well. So did my patient Cheryl, whose story I told in the beginning of this chapter. She suffered not only from MS but also from digestive issues characteristic of a condition known as leaky gut syndrome. Our intestinal lining contains more than four thousand square feet of surface area—bigger than most houses. When the lining is working right, it forms a barrier that controls what gets absorbed into the bloodstream. But when the lining develops tears or holes—usually from an overgrowth of unhealthy bacteria in your gastrointestinal tract, a high-sugar diet, or stress—it lets partially digested food, toxins, and bacteria leak out, leading to dangerous inflammation that plays a role in neurodegenerative brain disorders.

An unhealthy gut microbiome has been shown to contribute to everything from gastrointestinal disorders like leaky gut, celiac disease, and irritable bowel syndrome to autoimmune diseases like MS, as well as chronic fatigue syndrome, autism, fibromyalgia, arthritis, obesity, and mental illness. A number of problems can cause an imbalance in gut bacteria—frequent antibiotic use, excessive alcohol consumption, chronic stress, and a diet high in refined sugar, carbohydrates, and processed foods. But by avoiding sugar and grains and feeding your gastrointestinal tract the nutritious fats, healthy veggies, wild-caught fish, grass-fed meats, bone broth, and fermented foods found in my keto diet program, you can restore a healthy balance of bacteria. As inflammation calms, your gut begins to communicate "stand-down" signals to the brain—and your entire system comes into better balance.

Indeed, as Cheryl's MS symptoms improved, so did her gastrointestinal problems. But in order to achieve that kind of powerful result, you have to do keto the right way. Eating bacon and butter won't transform leaky gut or brain-related problems. In order to reap the full benefits, you need to give your body the highest-quality fat, protein, veggies, and fruit so you can diminish inflammation, promote the growth of health-giving gastrointestinal bacteria, and allow your gut and brain to heal.

THE ELEVEN BRAIN-PROTECTING SUPPLEMENTS THAT WORK SYNERGISTICALLY WITH KETOSIS

While diet alone will go a long way toward restoring and protecting your brain health, certain supplements can bolster the diet's effects on the brain and enhance your keto-brain experience. In addition to herbs and nutrients, nootropics can also help optimize your brain function. If you suffer from a brain-related condition, it's a good idea to consider supporting my keto diet program with brain-boosting supplements. Here are the top natural supplements that have beneficial effects on brain health:

Turmeric. One of the most powerful disease fighters on the planet, this renowned golden herb is the subject of more than ten thousand peer-reviewed studies. It comes from the *Curcuma longa* plant, which grows in India and other countries in Southeast Asia. Among its many effects is an ability to bolster the production of brain-derived neurotrophic factor (BDNF),[21] a protein that has been described as Miracle-Gro for the brain. Probably because of its effect on BDNF, turmeric has been shown to relieve depression. In a study reported in *Phytotherapy Research*, sixty people with depression were split into three groups.[22] One took Prozac, a commonly prescribed antidepressant, another took curcumin (the active substance in turmeric), and a third took both. After six weeks, the researchers found that curcumin was as effective as Prozac in improving depression; those taking both showed slightly greater improvement, but it wasn't even enough to be statistically significant. You can use turmeric in your cooking or take a supplement with 250 to 500 milligrams once or twice a day.

Resveratrol. The phytonutrient resveratrol, found in the skin of red grapes, red wine, raw cocoa, and dark berries like lingonberries, blueberries, and mulberries, affects your body on a cellular level. It's unique among antioxidants in that it can cross the blood-brain barrier, where it can offer vital protection against free radical damage and death. In addition, studies conducted at the Brain Performance and Nutrition Research Centre at Northumbria University in the United Kingdom showed that resveratrol increased blood flow to the brain[23]— an effect that could bolster healthy brain function and protect neurons as well. On my keto diet plan you need to limit most dietary sources of resveratrol, like blueberries, lingonberries and red wine, so I recommend using a supplement; take 500 milligrams a day.

Nootropics like citicoline, ashwagandha, and egg yolk extract. As I explained in Chapter 5, nootropics are cognitive enhancers that can improve your brain function, memory, creativity, and motivation. The formulation of these supplements varies by brand, so follow the standard dosage on the bottle.

Acai berry powder. Made from small, deep-purple acai berries native to Central and South America, especially Brazil, where they grow in parts of the Amazon rain forest, acai powder is chock-full of electrolytes, trace minerals, amino acids, and even small amounts of essential fatty acids. But its brain-bolstering power comes from its claim to fame as one of the most potent antioxidants in nature. The concentration of antioxidants in acai is believed to be ten times greater than that in red grapes. Add 1 scoop per day to your morning coffee or green juice.

CBD oil. Although cannabis oil (derived cannabidiol), a nonpsychoactive ingredient in marijuana plants, has been used in medicine for millennia, concern over the dangers of abuse led to its ban in the United States in the 1930s. In recent years, the medical community has begun taking a second look at this oil and acknowledged its potent effects on health, especially brain health. Research shows that CBD has a pharmacological profile similar to some atypical antipsychotic drugs, and studies have shown it can be helpful for psychosis and schizophrenia. In addition, CBD can reduce anxiety. It has been shown to provide relief to people with social anxiety disorder and may help with panic disorder, obsessive-compulsive disorder, and post-traumatic stress disorder.[24] It can also be an effective treatment for children suffering from seizure disorders who don't respond to traditional medications—in some cases offering complete relief to children who had been suffering hundreds of seizures a day. You can use CBD oil only if you live in a state where medical marijuana is legal. States vary in what they require to get a prescription to use medical cannabis. Because CBD oils aren't standardized, you'll need to talk to your doctor or the dispensary about dosage.

Omega-3 fatty acids. In addition to their impressive effects on heart health, omega-3 fatty acids have been shown to help with depression, anxiety, ADHD, schizophrenia, bipolar disorder, and Alzheimer's. One study on depression found that an omega-3 supplement was as effective in combatting the illness as antidepressant medication.[25] The reason these diet-derived fats are so healthy for the brain: The two fatty acids they contain—EPA and DHA—are components of cell membranes and are known for their ability to fight inflammation. Eat two or more 3.5-ounce servings of fatty fish, like salmon or tuna, per week and take a daily supplement containing 500 milligrams of EPA and DHA.

Collagen powder. This wonderful antiaging supplement has effects on skin, hair, and nails—and can also protect and soothe the lining of the digestive tract. As a result, it can be beneficial for those with gastrointestinal problems that may also play a role in brain health, like leaky gut syndrome, irritable bowel syndrome, Crohn's disease, and ulcerative colitis. Increased collagen intake strengthens and normalizes mucous membranes in the gastrointestinal lining and helps patch holes and tears that can lead to chronic inflammation. Add 1 scoop to your favorite keto beverage once or twice a day.

Lion's mane mushrooms. These crazy-looking fungi are well-known nootropics and are popular in traditional Chinese medicine. One study published in the *Journal of Agricultural and Food Chemistry* reported that lion's mane mushrooms not only offer neuroprotection but also improve anxiety, cognitive function, and depression.[26] One way they affect brain function is by enhancing the growth of axons and dendrites—the parts of brain cells that meet at the synapse (the space between cells), allowing intercellular communication. That could potentially help slow or reverse cell degeneration in the brain that occurs with diseases like Alzheimer's and Parkinson's. In one study, lion's mane mushroom was found to improve memory in mice with and without Alzheimer's,[27] and in another, it eased cognitive impairment in humans.[28] You might be able to find these mushrooms in Asian markets. If you can't, take a supplement and follow dosage directions on the bottle.

Rosemary oil. Extracted from the flowering tops and leaves of the small, fragrant evergreen plant, rosemary oil has been known to strengthen cognitive capacity for thousands of years. Researchers in the United Kingdom found that rosemary oil aromatherapy enhanced memory and alertness.[29] Mix 3 drops of rosemary oil with ½ teaspoon of coconut oil and rub it on your neck, or diffuse it for 1 hour a day.

Ginkgo biloba. Used medically in China for eons, ginkgo biloba has been widely studied for its anti-inflammatory, antioxidant, and circulation-boosting effects. Research shows that ginkgo can bolster concentration and reduce fatigue. When researchers at the University of Munich tested ginkgo against placebo on healthy adults' mental performance for four weeks, they found that the group taking ginkgo had better motor performance and emotional health.[30] There's also evidence that it can help people experiencing dementia-related cognitive decline, as well as those recovering from strokes and traumatic brain injuries. At the same time, because ginkgo is an adaptogen that helps your body cope with stress, it might bolster mood in those who struggle with depression and anxiety. Ginkgo is available in capsule, tablet, and liquid extract form, and standard dosages vary from 40 to 360 milligrams daily, so follow the directions on the bottle.

Probiotics, like kefir, fermented vegetables, and apple cider vinegar. Probiotics are the good bacteria that line your digestive tract and support your body's ability to absorb nutrients, fight infection, reduce inflammation, and keep you healthy as you age. Probiotics have been called "psychobiotics" because of their ability to positively impact brain function by lowering inflammation. They also produce vitamin B_{12}, the nutrient many modern diets are missing. B_{12} helps maintain the health of nerve cells, including those needed for neurotransmitter signaling. In other words, this missing vitamin affects your mood, energy level, and memory.

A healthy gut has a balance of good and bad bacteria—about 85 percent good and 15 percent bad—but the food you eat affects that ratio. A high-sugar, high-carb, heavily processed diet tips the scales toward the bad bacteria, creating "dysbiosis," or microbial imbalance, which fuels inflammation and puts you at risk of all sorts of illness, including MS, depression, anxiety, and others that affect your brain. Historically, we had plenty of probiotics in our diet from eating fresh foods from healthy soil, along with the fermented foods we talked about in Chapter 4. On my keto diet plan, you'll add those foods back into your everyday menu, which will give your good bacteria the opportunity to flourish. I encourage you to embrace the "power of sour" by eating foods that are teeming with powerful gut- and brain-protecting probiotics. It's one of the most effective ways I've found to protect your system's delicate internal bacterial balance and upgrade your cognitive processing from so-so to keto-brain. In addition to eating probiotic-rich foods, I recommend that you take a supplement containing 50 billion CFU one or two times a day.

We all want to shield our brains from damage and preserve our intellectual fitness—and the truth about how carbs and sugar can undermine the health of your cognitive machinery is alarming. As psychiatrist Georgia Ede said in a post on PsychologyToday.com: "If you have a brain, you need to know about ketogenic diets."[31] She's right. And my keto diet program offers a powerful two-prong approach to protection: By eliminating carbs, it shelters you from the most dangerous ingredients in the modern diet, and by increasing your daily consumption of healthy fats and healing greens and herbs, it gives your brain the nutrients it needs to stay keen, engaged, and on point for the rest of your life.

CHAPTER 9

Ketosis Is a Hero for Hormones

The Diet That Can Help Balance Estrogen, Testosterone, Thyroid, and More

When I met thirty-year-old Miriam, she was forty pounds over-weight, her posture was slumped as if she couldn't muster the energy to hold her body upright, and she looked tired. I wasn't surprised when she told me she'd been diagnosed with hypothyroidism, or low thyroid, which causes fatigue and weight gain. She also had polycystic ovary syndrome (PCOS), a hormonal disorder that strikes an estimated 10 percent of women of reproductive age[1] (but may actually be far more common) and causes a constellation of symptoms, including weight gain, infertility, irregular periods, fatigue, moodiness, insomnia, acne, and facial hair.

Miriam's doctor had recommended a low-fat diet to get her weight under control and prescribed medication to bolster her thyroid hormone level. When those strategies failed to help her lose weight or improve her energy, she went to a naturopathic doctor who recommended B_{12} shots, which help with energy, and suggested she start eating organic produce and meats. Miriam began feeling a little more vital. But she still struggled with frequent fatigue, she wasn't losing weight—and she worried she'd be on medication for the rest of her life.

I listened to her history, then proposed a different approach. I told her my goal was not to treat the PCOS or the thyroid disorder but rather to cure the *root cause* of both those hormonal problems. I explained to her that hormones are chemical messengers, and they work in concert, affecting one another in important ways. Some hormones' sole responsibility is producing more of another hormone! Hormones also affect every cell and function in your body. They regulate your metabolism, your hunger and thirst, your interest in sex, your ability to become pregnant, your energy, your sleep cycle, your immune system, your response to stress, and your emotions and mood.

Each type of hormone is stored and produced in a certain gland, like the ovaries, testicles, thyroid, pancreas, or adrenals, to name a few. In response to a signal from the brain, the thyroid, say, secretes thyroid hormone into the blood, which carries it to the cells in the body with receptors designed to respond to its particular chemical signal. In some cases, you can treat a hormonal problem in isolation. But that approach can be like replacing one violinist and expecting the whole orchestra to improve.

In order to make more global, lasting changes in people's health, you need to affect the conductor of the orchestra, and if there's one way to do that, it's by focusing on insulin. This pivotal hormone, which runs amok when you eat a sugar- and carb-heavy diet, affects everything else. I suspected Miriam's cells had become insulin resistant, causing her blood levels of glucose and insulin to become elevated. (A reminder about how this works: After a meal, the pancreas secretes insulin, which takes sugar out of your blood and transports it to the cells in your muscles and brain to use as fuel. But when your body is insulin resistant, your cells become less responsive to insulin's efforts, so less glucose gets into your cells and more stays your blood; as a result, your pancreas makes more insulin, exacerbating the problem.)

I also wanted to tone down Miriam's stress response, because I believed her adrenal glands, which secrete adrenaline and are involved in the fight-or-flight system, weren't functioning properly. And I wanted to improve the health of the microbes in her gut—another way to transform whole-body health. To that end, I put her on a ketogenic diet to rein in insulin and support adrenal function and healthy digestion. I also prescribed probiotics to rebuild a wholesome population of bacteria in her gut and suggested she take ashwagandha for stress and B complex, which has a range of B vitamins, in place of the B_{12} shots for energy.

From the perspective of traditional Chinese medicine, PCOS is caused by excess dampness in the body, along with a deficiency of qi, or energy, in the kidneys and spleen. Foods that are bitter help dry up dampness, so I recommended that she consume asparagus, arugula, celery, radishes, parsley, pumpkin, and onion—then support her qi with both astragalus and ashwagandha.

After four months she lost thirty-five pounds, and by six months she had lost all forty. Her thyroid hormones normalized, and she was able to completely stop taking her thyroid medication. She felt so energetic she began walking regularly, then advanced to group fitness classes three times a week. Even better: Within six months she was pregnant. By giving her body lots of healthy fat and virtually eliminating carbs, we were able to get Miriam's insulin under control, which helped all her other hormones fall into line.

Thanks to its positive influence on insulin, the ketogenic diet can have a robust effect on a variety of hormone-related issues, including PMS, menopause-related symptoms, infertility, and low testosterone. Here's what the latest compelling science has revealed about keto's ability to alleviate these disorders and create an environment in which your hormones are able to work more harmoniously and your health is restored.

POLYCYSTIC OVARY SYNDROME

It's no surprise that Miriam responded well to the ketogenic diet. PCOS is driven by an imbalance in a number of hormones that not only interfere with ovulation but also promote insulin resistance. For instance, women with PCOS don't ovulate, because they have too little follicle-stimulating hormone (FSH), so their eggs don't mature, and too much luteinizing hormone (LH), which stimulates the production of androgens (male hormones, like testosterone), contributing to insulin resistance and interfering with ovulation. As a result, the eggs remain in the ovaries and form small cysts, a condition that worsens month after month.

At the same time, sufferers have low levels of sex-hormone-binding globuline (SHBG), a condition that can drive insulin resistance; insulin resistance can lower levels of SHBG as well. SHBG's job is to bind to free testosterone in the blood so the male hormone isn't able to affect the cells in women's bodies. But when SHBG is low, levels of free testosterone rise, pushing insulin resistance even higher (and interfering with ovulation).

In women with PCOS, the combination of high free testosterone and low SHBG sets up a vicious cycle: It increases insulin resistance and promotes fat storage in the belly around the liver and pancreas—and excess "visceral fat," as it's called, promotes insulin resistance and inflammation and stimulates the production of *more* male hormones, which further impairs the cells' ability to respond to insulin.

My keto diet program's high-fat, low-carb profile effectively breaks the dangerous cycle by taming insulin resistance and burning fat more quickly than any other dietary approach. In a small study reported in *Nutrition & Metabolism*, obese women who had been diagnosed with PCOS followed a ketogenic diet for twenty-four weeks.[2] By the end of the study, they had lost an average of 12 percent of their body weight, their free testosterone had dropped 22 percent, and their fasting insulin was down 54 percent. There was also a reduction in the women's LH/FSH ratio that, the researchers said, "may be indicative of endocrine re-normalization resulting from the low-carbohydrate ketogenic diet intervention, due to an improvement in insulin sensitivity"—results that echo an earlier study that found similar decreases in weight and insulin levels. What's more, two women in the study who had been struggling to conceive were able to get pregnant—evidence that the diet was able to turn around the core mechanisms of PCOS. (More on keto and fertility in the following section.)

While being in ketosis can help with insulin resistance, my keto diet's superhealthy ingredients can magnify that effect. Studies show that the high omega-3 fatty acid content of fish like wild-caught salmon and sardines may help lower insulin levels and improve insulin sensitivity in women with PCOS,[3] and walnuts may increase SHBG while almonds may reduce male hormone levels in sufferers.[4] Likewise, foods rich in lignans, like flaxseeds, sesame seeds, curly kale, broccoli, and cabbage, might reduce free testosterone. A case study in a thirty-one-year-old woman with PCOS found that eating 30 grams per day of flaxseeds significantly decreased testosterone levels.[5] It also makes sense to take a vitamin D supplement. Up to 85 percent of women with PCOS are thought to have a deficiency;[6] adding vitamin D might improve insulin sensitivity, support weight loss, slow the formation of ovarian cysts, and minimize both inflammation and androgen levels.

INFERTILITY

I've seen patients who have struggled with infertility become pregnant after starting a ketogenic diet. I remember one patient, Elizabeth, who had been trying to get pregnant for four years before finally having success after switching to a high-fat, very-low-carb diet. The Internet is buzzing with stories from women who've had similar experiences. But what does the research say?

A review of studies looking at the effect of low-carbohydrate diets on fertility concluded that there is convincing evidence that reducing carbohydrates can lower circulating insulin levels, rebalance hormones, help infertile women resume healthy ovulation, and improve pregnancy rates.[7] Reducing insulin seems to be the key—and it helps with men's sperm counts, too, which is good news, considering that sperm counts in men in North America, Australia, Europe, and New Zealand have dropped by more than 50 percent in less than four decades.[8] A study that analyzed 189 men ages eighteen to twenty-two found that as carb intake and dietary glycemic load increased, sperm concentrations declined.[9] (Dietary glycemic load is a measure of how much the food you eat raises glucose levels—and the more glucose you have, the higher your insulin.)

A study at the Harvard School of Public Health followed 18,555 married, premenopausal women without a history of infertility over eight years as they tried to get pregnant.[10] During the follow-up, 438 of the women reported infertility caused by problems with ovulation—and the researchers found a correlation between the condition and high carbohydrate and sugar intake. Their book about the long-term study, *The Fertility Diet*, didn't specifically recommend the low-carb approach that I advocate, but it did suggest several dietary strategies that dovetail with the ketogenic diet, including avoiding simple carbs and sugar, using more monounsaturated and polyunsaturated fats to improve the body's sensitivity to insulin, and choosing whole-fat dairy products.

Weight loss itself is beneficial for fertility, and there's no better way to shed weight than through my keto diet program. Being overweight or obese is strongly related to poor semen quality, and women who are obese have higher rates of ovulatory problems and miscarriages than normal-weight women. Similarly, type 2 diabetes is associated with fertility issues, and the ketogenic diet is effective for improving glycemic control and promoting weight loss in people with diabetes.

When you're trying to get pregnant, it's important to get plenty of iron from plant sources like spinach and beets, take a multivitamin with 400 micrograms of folic acid (ideally methylated folic acid), and eat folate-rich foods, like green leafy vegetables. Both men and women should eat organic foods and wild-caught fish, because food that contains pesticides and other hormones can have a negative effect on your body's hormones. And it's a good idea to eat more foods that are high in vitamin E, like almonds and spinach, and vitamin C, like strawberries, camu camu, broccoli, bell peppers, kale, parsley, and cauliflower.

Once you get pregnant, you should add more healthy carbs, like berries and beans, back into your diet to ensure you get a full range of nutrition, including folic acid and fiber, as well as sufficient carbs to maintain the healthy growth of the baby. Aim for a macronutrient profile of 55 percent fat, 20 percent protein, and 25 percent carbs.

PREMENSTRUAL SYNDROME

About 75 percent of women suffer from premenstrual symptoms,[11] like headaches, moodiness, bloating, breast tenderness, cramping, food craving, anxiety, and fatigue—and they range from mild to debilitating.

Considering that the average woman has 450 periods in her lifetime (triple the number in our ancestors, who died younger and spent more time pregnant and nursing), that can add up to a lot of agony. PMS usually starts in the days after ovulation, when estrogen and progesterone levels drop. The cause is likely related to declining hormones, but research shows that stress, thyroid problems, and environmental toxins seem to play a role as well.

My wife, Chelsea, was among the women who struggled every month with symptoms—until she switched from a nutritious, whole-foods diet to keto (specifically keto cycling). Her result was surprising, because she was already a health fanatic. But it showed me that my keto diet program holds benefits for PMS sufferers above and beyond what even the healthiest "traditional" diet can provide.

In general, we know that a sugar-heavy diet fuels the condition. Women with PMS eat 275 percent more refined sugar than nonsufferers, according to one study[12]—a finding that makes sense from a biological perspective. After you eat a meal high in sugar, insulin soars—and insulin can lower levels of SHBG, allowing both estrogen and testosterone to increase. With estrogen high, the delicate balance of estrogen and progesterone (a hormone that promotes well-being and a feeling of calm) is thrown off, causing insomnia, anxiety, and irritability—classic signs of PMS. The good news: On my keto diet plan, you'll gain control of raging insulin and reduce your monthly symptoms. It's also likely that you'll lose weight, and PMS is more common in women who are heavier. The ketogenic diet can also help reduce insulin-related inflammation, and inflammation drives PMS, as it has a negative impact on the liver, the organ that is responsible for eliminating excess estrogen from your system.

My keto diet plan will protect you from this monthly burden in a number of other ways. Women with PMS typically are not getting enough of certain key nutrients, including calcium, B vitamins (especially B_6), vitamins K and E, and magnesium—all of which are plentiful in the keto diet.

Because PMS can cause gastrointestinal disturbances, you should eat at least 30 grams of fiber every day from foods like chia seeds, flaxseeds, collard greens, kale, spinach, broccoli, avocados, raspberries, and blackberries. Leafy greens are also great sources of fiber as well as calcium, magnesium, and vitamin K. Fiber helps maintain proper hormone balance by binding to estrogen and carrying it out of the body.

You'll be eating lots of healthy fat on my keto diet program, but if you suffer from PMS, make sure you're getting two types in particular: omega-3 fats, like wild-caught salmon, sardines, and anchovies, which help reduce pain and inflammation, and the unsaturated fat in avocados. Eating an avocado a day naturally balances hormones, because it's high not only in healthy fat but also in fiber, magnesium, potassium, and vitamin B_6.

I also recommend two adaptogenic herbs—ashwagandha and holy basil, which have been shown to reduce the stress hormone cortisol, balance hormones, and minimize symptoms of PMS. Reducing stress is critical. In one study, women who reported high stress levels prior to ovulation were twenty-five times more likely to have PMS symptoms.[13] The reason: When cortisol rises, it throws off your hormone balance.

If you know you have an imbalance of estrogen, the herb vitex (also known as chasteberry) has been shown to be effective for reducing symptoms of PMS. Dong quai, another Chinese herb, may relieve PMS symptoms too, since it's high in iron and builds healthy blood. (Just don't use it if you have heavy periods or are pregnant, because it can cause extra bleeding.) Formulations vary, so follow dosage directions on the bottle.

Finally, try mixing 2 drops of clary sage oil with 1 tablespoon of a carrier oil, like almond oil, and rubbing it on your lower abdomen. Apply a warm compress to the area for 2 to 5 minutes. Clary sage is a natural hormone balancer and can reduce symptoms.

MENOPAUSE

The transition into menopause can be tough for many women. With symptoms that affect 75 percent of women,[14] like mood swings, fatigue, declining sex drive, unexplained weight gain, and hot flashes that can strike out of the blue during the day and often interrupt sleep, it's a challenging time of life. Nearly half of women between ages forty-five and sixty-four have trouble sleeping, according to a National Sleep Foundation survey.

As with PMS, you can chalk up these symptoms to changing hormones. At least a decade before you have your last menstrual cycle, estrogen, testosterone, progesterone, and dehydroepiandrosterone (DHEA) begin fluctuating and triggering symptoms—a time known as perimenopause. For instance, as estrogen wanes, it disrupts the functioning of the part of your brain's hypothalamus that controls body temperature and regulates other automatic processes, like hunger, thirst, and sleep.

Again, my keto diet program attacks the problem from several angles. The abundance of healthy fats you're eating when you do keto right promotes the absorption of fat-soluble vitamins, including vitamin D, which contributes to the production of sex hormones, including estrogen and testosterone—and that helps support not only a healthy libido but also energy and mood. Since most people's D levels drop as they age, getting more through your diet is important. At the same time, fueling your body with ketones instead of glucose helps stabilize your energy and create more ideal conditions for sleep.

When Mayo Clinic researchers had women with hot flashes eat 1.5 ounces of flaxseed daily for six weeks, they found the average number of hot flashes dropped by half and their severity plummeted 57 percent.[15] Study participants also said their mood improved and they had fewer unusual symptoms, like joint and muscle pain, sweating, and chills. Flaxseed helps because it's high in phytoestrogens (essentially estrogen from plants), like lignans.

During menopause it's important to focus on a keto alkaline diet. As I explained in Chapter 3, that means eating lots of green, leafy veggies and adding a scoop of a powdered greens supplement to your favorite keto-friendly beverage every day. An alkaline diet optimizes insulin, cortisol, and other hormones that contribute to menopause symptoms, including hot flashes. Consuming too many acidic foods creates chronic low-grade acidosis, which depletes precious minerals like magnesium, calcium, and potassium from the body and increases inflammation.

Add these three menopause-easing herbs to your diet, too:

Ginseng may bolster mood and enhance well-being and have a positive effect on other symptoms, like hot flashes. Take 1 gram daily, or 500 milligrams twice a day.

Black cohosh has been used in TCM for thousands of years to improve the symptoms of menopause. Take 80 milligrams one or two times a day.

Licorice root has also proven to be effective for reducing the frequency and severity of hot flashes. You shouldn't take licorice root if you have heart, liver, or kidney issues, however, because glycyrrhizin, which gives the plant its sweetness, can increase blood pressure and reduce potassium levels. If you don't have one of those conditions, take 6 grams a day.

SEXUAL DYSFUNCTION

Lack of libido is common in both men and women. A variety of factors can affect sex drive, including stress, depression, relationship strife, prescription medications, and alcohol or drug use, but two biggies that the ketogenic diet can help with are hormonal issues and body image problems due to excess weight.

Low testosterone can play a role in declining libido in both genders. Women's testosterone levels peak in their mid-twenties and steadily decline through menopause, when levels of estrogen start dropping as well. Men's begin to drop with age as well. And here's what's interesting: Studies have shown that women on low-fat diets experience a significant reduction in estrogen,[16] which can lead to both reduced sex drive and challenging symptoms like vaginal dryness.

A small study also found that when men ate a higher-fat diet, their testosterone levels increased[17] — and low-fat diets have been shown to do the opposite.[18] I saw this in one of my patients, Jim. He was a successful entrepreneur and father, but he confided in me that he was struggling with erectile dysfunction. I laid out a keto eating plan for him and suggested he start lifting weights. When I saw him two months later, he had lost twenty-five pounds, he'd started cycling regularly as well as strength training, and, he said happily, his erectile dysfunction had disappeared.

My keto diet plan can revive your libido by helping you lose weight as well. You'll feel more confident about your body. But there are physiological mechanisms at play when you're overweight that have a negative impact on sex drive as well. For instance, one study found that men who are heavier are more likely to experience erectile dysfunction.[19]

To get the most libido-boosting power out of my keto diet, you can also supplement with hormone-supporting herbs and supplements. For men, ginseng, deer antler, fenugreek, and zinc have been used for thousands of years to support testosterone production. And for women, vitex, dong quai, and codonopsis can naturally support a healthy libido. For both men and women with libido deficiency, epimedium and tribulus also work well. Formulations vary, so follow dosages on bottles.

THYROID HEALTH

You might have heard that the ketogenic diet can have an adverse affect on thyroid health, which would be bad—if it were accurate. The truth is more complicated. Your thyroid produces hormones that influence dozens of vital functions in your body, from energy and metabolism to body temperature and heart rate. There are three main hormones you need to understand to grasp how the thyroid functions. Thyroid-stimulating hormone, or TSH, is produced by the pituitary gland in the brain and stimulates the production of the other two players, triiodothyronine (T3) and thyroxine (T4). T4 is the main hormone produced by the thyroid gland. It travels through the blood to your liver, where it's converted into T3, the active form of the hormone that sends instructions to every cell in your body.

The term "hypothyroid," or low thyroid, means you're low in T4 and TSH—a condition that can cause weight gain, hair loss, fatigue, impaired memory, and difficulty staying warm. It's an autoimmune condition that's fueled by inflammation. Lowering inflammation can help with low thyroid by improving the conversion of T4 to T3—so that's one mechanism by which the ketogenic diet is helpful. Likewise, the fluctuating blood sugar that occurs on a high-carb diet contributes to the formation of inflammatory proteins called advanced glycolytic enzymes that may inhibit thyroid production; by burning ketones for fuel instead of glucose, you eliminate this inflammation pathway as well. Finally, insulin resistance from being overweight and eating a high-carb diet blocks the conversion of the inactive T4 to the active T3; on my keto diet plan, glucose isn't an issue.

Still, there's some evidence that when you lose weight on any diet, including the ketogenic diet, your levels of T3 drop. Theoretically, you're more likely to experience the symptoms of hypothyroidism, but here's the thing: Most of my patients don't. We don't really know why. But a study in the *Journal of the American Medical Association* found that in overweight and obese young adults who lost 10 to 15 percent of their body weight, those consuming a low-fat diet had the greatest decrease in metabolic rate.[20] Metabolic rate, which is controlled by the thyroid, dropped the least with a very-low-carb diet. It could be that nutritional ketosis improves the function of your cells and the mitochondria, or energy factories, so they're more responsive to T3 and able to function perfectly fine on lower levels of the hormone.

In any case, the smartest way to approach thyroid issues on a ketogenic diet is to pay attention to how you feel. If you're sluggish and tired and struggling to lose weight, you might need to skip to keto cycling and throw intermittent carb days into the mix. The best carbohydrates for those with thyroid conditions are berries and sprouted rice that is high in GABA (also known as germinated rice).

In addition, eat plenty of these foods that support the thyroid:

Selenium, which helps balance out T4 production in the body. Good sources are yellowfin tuna, canned sardines, grass-fed beef, beef liver, eggs, and spinach.

B vitamins, particularly thiamine and B_{12}. Thiamine is found in asparagus, sesame seeds, pistachios, herring, cremini mushrooms, ground flaxseed, and spinach. Good sources of B_{12} include grass-fed beef, tuna, raw cheese, cottage cheese, lamb, eggs, and salmon.

Probiotics like kefir, cultured veggies, coconut kefir, natto, probiotic yogurt, kvass, and raw cheese. Leaky gut has been linked to hypothyroidism, so eating these foods can restore the health of your gut microbes and help treat the illness from the inside out. It also makes sense to take 50 billion CFU of a probiotic supplement once or twice a day.

Proteolytic enzymes reduce inflammation. If you have an autoimmune-related thyroid condition like Hashimoto's disease, taking proteolytic enzymes like bromelain can reduce inflammation of the thyroid. Supplement with 500 to 800 milligrams of bromelain every day.

Ashwagandha is good for healing the thyroid and can be consumed in capsules, tea, or tincture form. It helps you adapt to and deal with stress. In studies it has been shown to aid both underactive and overactive thyroid. In addition to ashwagandha, herbs used in traditional Chinese medicine to improve thyroid function include rehmannia and bacopa. Dosages vary by formulation, so follow instructions on the bottle.

ADRENAL HEALTH

As I explained in Chapter 6, your adrenal glands release the stress hormone cortisol in the morning to help you wake up and during times when you're experiencing stress. But in our overstressed culture, many people's adrenal glands are overtaxed. Their bodies are constantly churning out cortisol in response to the daily demands. Besieged by this constant stimulation, they develop "adrenal fatigue," a condition in which the adrenals stop producing hormones efficiently. In addition to an overload of cortisol, people with adrenal fatigue often don't have enough DHEA, the "parent hormone" responsible for the creation of many other vital hormones. The condition, which causes brain fog, hair loss, hormone imbalance, decreased libido, sleep disturbances, insulin resistance, and weight gain, isn't endorsed by mainstream medicine but has long been recognized by practitioners of traditional Chinese medicine.

High cortisol makes your cells more resistant to insulin, so a diet that reduces insulin can be one prong in an effective approach to treatment. The idea is to remove any foods that tax your adrenals, including caffeine, sugar and sweeteners, carbohydrates, processed foods, and hydrogenated oils. What you're left with is the nutrient-dense, low-carb, high-fiber foods that form the basis of my keto diet program: olives, avocados, cruciferous vegetables, fatty fish like wild-caught salmon, free-range chicken and turkey, bone broth, nuts, seeds, fermented foods, and medicinal mushrooms, like cordyceps.

In addition to getting seven to eight hours of sleep and minimizing stress however you can — with yoga, meditation, prayer, laughter, or time with close friends — you also should support your adrenals with herbs, spices, and essential oils. Here are the ten I recommend:

Adaptogenic herbs like rhodiola, schisandra, ashwagandha, ginseng, codonopsis, and holy basil. Research indicates that adaptogenic herbs can lower cortisol levels and mediate your stress response. Dosages vary, so follow instructions on the bottle.

Licorice root is available in extract form. It helps increase DHEA, the parent hormone. As I mentioned previously, you should avoid licorice root if you have heart, liver, or kidney issues. Otherwise, you can take 6 grams a day.

Omega-3 fatty acids. Their ability to counter insulin resistance and inflammation offers helpful support for the adrenals. Eat two or more 3.5-ounce servings of fatty fish, like salmon or tuna, per week and take a daily supplement containing 500 milligrams of EPA and DHA.

Magnesium can support healthy sleep, and many people in the United States are deficient. Load up on healthy sources of magnesium, like spinach, Swiss chard, and avocado, and take a daily supplement with 300 milligrams.

B-complex vitamins play a crucial role in the stress response. Many people are deficient in B_{12}, and people with adrenal stress are often low in B_5. Take a B-complex vitamin with 5 milligrams of B_5 and 2.4 micrograms of B_{12}.

Vitamin C is known as a stress-busting nutrient that helps your body bounce back from taxing emotional experiences. Since you're eating fewer fruits high in vitamin C on the keto diet, it's a good idea to supplement, especially if you're struggling with adrenal fatigue. Men should take 90 milligrams a day and women should take 75; pregnant and breastfeeding women should take 85 and 120 milligrams a day, respectively.

Vitamin D has been shown in preliminary research to have a positive impact on adrenal function. Sitting in the sun for twenty minutes without sunscreen will help bolster your levels, but it's a good idea to supplement with up to 5,000 IU per day.

Selenium deficiency can negatively impact your adrenal glands, according to studies in animals. You can easily get enough of the mineral from my keto diet program. One medium egg, for instance, contains 146 micrograms, nearly three times the recommended daily amount of 55 micrograms for adults. It's also found in Brazil nuts, sunflower seeds, liver, tuna, chicken breast, salmon, and mushrooms.

Lavender oil has a calming effect and can reduce stress. Research has also suggested that it may lower cortisol levels when you inhale it as part of an aromatherapy protocol. Diffuse it while you work, add a few drops to a warm bath at night, or rub a dab on your temples, your wrists, and the soles of your feet.

Rosemary oil is an essential oil that can help reduce cortisol and oxidative stress on cells. Diffuse it into the air or add 1 or 2 drops to a glass of water and drink it.

Hormone-related conditions are usually treated with hormone replacement therapy, which can create additional problems and imbalances. But research on the keto diet shows that you can effectively support hormone health with food. By creating a curative environment and addressing the root cause of common hormone-related disorders, my keto diet program gives you a way to restore the natural, healthy functioning of these powerful chemicals so your body can heal itself.

CHAPTER 10

Keto the Cancer Killer

How Fueling Your Body with Ketones Attacks Cancer

Witnessing my mom beat cancer with a modified keto diet (about 60 percent fat, 30 percent protein, and 10 percent carbs), along with supportive lifestyle tactics that included affirmations, prayer, gentle movement, herbal remedies, and essential oils, was a pivotal moment in my evolution as a functional medicine doctor. It convinced me that by eating plenty of nutritious fat and healthy veggies and a moderate amount of clean protein—and at the same time radically reducing carbs—you can heal the body and even obliterate one of the most frightening and prevalent killers of our time. Since then I've heard any number of compelling stories about people using the ketogenic diet as part of a successful cancer treatment program. One comes from Jordan Rubin, my dear friend, mentor, and business partner.

In July 2008, Jordan developed discomfort in his abdomen. He thought he had a hernia—and his doctor agreed that was the most likely diagnosis. But during the exploratory surgery to repair the injury, they discovered that he actually had advanced testicular cancer that had spread to his lymph nodes.

Jordan was the last person you'd think would get cancer. He was thirty-two. He was in fantastic shape. He had a superhealthy diet of organic sprouted whole grains, organic fruits and vegetables, fermented dairy, grass-fed beef, and pastured eggs and poultry. He had written twenty books on health and was about to record a TV series on sports nutrition. His cancer developed because of a congenital abnormality. Even so, he was as stunned as anyone. But thanks to his in-depth knowledge of the way the body works, he felt confident he could conquer it.

"I'd already experienced the disease-fighting power of diet first-hand, because I'd beaten Crohn's disease with alternative practices. So I told my doctor I wanted to treat cancer naturally, too," recalls Jordan. "He looked at me and my wife and said, 'Don't blank with this. You have a one hundred percent chance of dying within ninety days if you don't get appropriate treatment.'"

Jordan and his wife had a four-year-old son, and they had just adopted two infants. He knew he needed to take an aggressive approach to tackling the disease. He was also convinced he could do it without chemotherapy or radiation. So he told his wife he wanted forty days to try it his way. If a follow-up CT scan revealed that the cancer was still raging, he'd consent to a more traditional approach.

"I had read about the ketogenic diet and understood that you could starve cancer cells by burning ketones instead of glucose for fuel, so the minute I got the diagnosis I knew that I wanted to go on a high-fat, nutrient-dense, low-carb, moderate-protein diet," he says.

He began eating "an astronomical amount" of healthy fat every day—several avocados, coconut meat, wild sockeye salmon ceviche, pastured eggs, and grass-fed bison cooked in olive oil and grass-fed butter—along with a quart of green juice made from celery, zucchini, parsley, cucumber, and raw cream or coconut cream, nutritious fat to help his body absorb the vegetables' nutrients. "I followed the principles of the keto diet, with an emphasis on nutrient-dense, raw foods," he says.

While food formed the cornerstone of Jordan's approach, he didn't rely on diet alone. His routine also included a sixty-minute essential oil massage, lymphatic drainage, a two-hour infrared sauna, acupuncture, deep breathing, forgiveness exercises, prayer, and meditation. "To keep my stress levels in check, I didn't tell many people about my cancer, because the intensity of other people's worry can be taxing," he says.

On the fortieth day, he went for a CT scan. A week later, he received the results he was looking for: His cancer had retreated.

That was ten years ago. "I'm forty-three now, and I still exercise avidly, coach my kids in Little League, and have a busy, thriving career," he says. "I eat the same way I did when my cancer was diagnosed, and I've become even more passionate about sharing the message of healthy fat. When your body runs on fat instead of glucose, not only do you starve cancer cells, but the fat also absorbs toxins and carries them out of your system. With traditional cancer treatment, the goal is to kill the cancer before you waste away. With the ketogenic diet, I did the opposite. I fed myself an abundance of calories and nutrition and allowed my body to get rid of the cancer on its own."

In the decade since Jordan was first diagnosed, there's been an explosion of research on the ketogenic diet and cancer. Scientists are beginning to drill down on the types for which it's most effective, as well as whether it can be beneficial as an adjunct to conventional chemo and radiation (early evidence is positive)—and whether it might be helpful in preventing cancer in the first place (there are hopeful signs it can).

These compelling studies, as well as the success stories I've heard from family and friends, have deepened my conviction that the ketogenic diet has remarkable cancer-fighting ability. It's more than a diet. Using fat as fuel is potentially a way to fend off cancer as well as battle it once it takes hold. It has immense untapped potential for the field of oncology as well as for anyone who has been diagnosed with this deadly disease.

THE BIOLOGY OF CANCER — AND WHY THE KETOGENIC DIET CAN HELP

Cancer is the second leading cause of death in the United States, falling just behind heart disease. It kills more people than stroke, Alzheimer's, diabetes, the flu, pneumonia, kidney disease, and accidents *combined*.[1] Even with recent advances in pharmaceutical treatments and surgical approaches, cancer is still a menace—which is why interest in using a ketogenic diet to fight the disease is growing.

Cancer cells aren't like any other cells in your body. They need glucose to proliferate and thrive. While healthy cells can run on ketones or glucose, cancer cells rely almost exclusively on glucose—and they need a lot of it. To maintain their rapid multiplication and survival, they use twenty times more glucose than normal cells. So when you eliminate carbs, you eliminate their go-to fuel source.

In the 1920s, Otto Warburg, a German doctor and Nobel laureate, discovered that cancer cells alter the way they metabolize glucose to support their frenetic growth. When you're eating carbs, the mitochondria in healthy cells use oxygen to break down glucose and turn it into ATP, the molecules the body uses for energy. The process, known as aerobic glycolysis (because it uses oxygen), produces thirty-two molecules of ATP for every molecule of glucose. Cancer cells, however, use anaerobic glycolysis, a less efficient approach (it produces only about two molecules of ATP for every molecule of glucose) but a far speedier one that churns out ATP almost one hundred times faster than normal cells.

The metabolic differences between healthy cells and tumor cells have been traced to dysfunctional mitochondria—and they are so striking that some scientists are now starting to think of cancer as a metabolic disease that is the result of the unique structure and function of mutated cells' mitochondria.

Cancer cells' reliance on large amounts of glucose, and glucose alone, is their most notable weakness, and the ketogenic diet offers a simple, risk-free way to exploit it. By taking this carbohydrate-related fuel off the table and feeding your body with ketones, the ketogenic diet effectively cuts off cancer cells' food supply, so they stop proliferating, wither, and sometimes even die.

In studies of animals with tumors, the survival of animals whose calories are restricted, which can force them to use ketones instead of glucose for fuel, is significantly prolonged compared to that of animals that are fed normally.[2] In 1962, there was a report in the scientific literature of two patients with metastatic tumors who were cured when they were put in a hypoglycemic (low-blood-sugar) coma.[3] Likewise, high blood sugar is a predictor of poor survival in patients with a variety of types of cancer[4] and has been correlated with an increased risk of developing cancer of the esophagus, pancreas, liver, colon, rectum, stomach, and prostate.[5]

That's not surprising when you understand what glucose does to your body. When you eat a typical high-carb meal and experience an elevation in blood glucose, it impairs the transport of ascorbic acid, or vitamin C, into immune cells—and vitamin C is necessary for the immune system to effectively respond to malignant cells. Even more dangerous, high blood sugar prompts insulin to rise, which stimulates the release of pro-inflammatory cytokines, like interleukin-6 (IL-6), that fuel cancer progression.

By now you know that burning fat for fuel effectively slashes your insulin production. By doing so, it may also slow tumor growth, not just because insulin triggers pro-inflammatory cytokines but because insulin is an "anabolic" hormone, meaning it makes cells grow—both healthy cells and cancerous ones. Indeed, a study in *Cancer Research* found that mice with cancer consuming a low-carb diet had lower levels of both glucose and insulin—and significantly slower tumor growth—compared to mice eating a carb-heavy Western diet.[6]

Reducing glucose and insulin through carbohydrate reduction might also protect you from developing cancer in the first place. Research has shown, for instance, that women with a high sugar intake are at increased risk of developing breast cancer. A study of nearly three thousand women on Long Island, half of whom had been diagnosed with breast cancer, found that those with the highest intake of sweets were at greater risk of breast cancer than those with lower intakes[7]—results that are consistent with other studies that implicate insulin in the development of breast cancer. Another paper in *BMC Public Health* found that sweet foods and sugar-sweetened beverages were associated with higher breast density,[8] a risk factor for breast cancer.

Likewise, a study of 566 men in the Uppsala Longitudinal Study of Adult Men in Sweden found that those who adhered to a low-carb diet had a lower risk of developing prostate cancer[9]—lending credence to the idea that cutting carbs can be protective. Other studies show that high glucose and high insulin levels are both predictors of cancer occurrence and cancer-related mortality.

There may even be something about ketones themselves that's beneficial. In a study in the *International Journal of Cancer*, researchers looked at the behavior of tumor cells in a petri dish as well as in adult mice.[10] They fed the mice a standard diet supplemented with one of two things: 1,3-butanediol, a supplement that the body converts into beta-hydroxybutyrate (BHB), one of the main ketones the body uses as fuel; or a supplement of ketone ester, a raw form of BHB. What they found: Both supplements decreased proliferation and viability of the cancer cells in the mice, even though they were also getting lots of glucose in their diets—and prolonged the mice's survival by 51 percent (with the 1,3-butanediol) and 69 percent (with the ketone ester). The supplements elicited anticancer effects in the lab samples as well.

Research on employing the ketogenic diet as a therapy for cancer is still relatively new. Not all types of cancer have been studied, and scientists are still trying to clarify the ins and outs of how and why it's effective. But diet is a low-risk intervention compared to most traditional cancer treatments. Moreover, many mainstream cancer therapies are designed to exploit the weaknesses of cancer cells, just as the ketogenic diet does. There's a lot left to learn, but there's a clear, plausible biological basis for why a high-fat, low-carb diet can weaken cancer cells' ability to grow and spread, and that's drawing increasing interest from a broad range of researchers and clinicians. Here's what science has revealed so far about how the ketogenic diet can be helpful for treating four common types of cancer.

Brain cancer

The ketogenic diet has been most widely studied in malignant glioma, the primary type of brain tumor. It's difficult to treat, especially in its most frequent and aggressive form, glioblastoma multiforme, which has a poor prognosis, with a median survival of twelve to fifteen months from the time of diagnosis. Malignant glioma cells, like those of many cancers, depend on glucose to grow and survive, so they're a good target for the keto diet. And alternative treatments are desperately needed, since there are concerns within the medical community that the current therapeutic approaches, like surgery and chemo, might actually drive tumor progression by causing tissue injury that leads to inflammation.[11] In addition, glucocorticoids, a type of steroid that reduces inflammation, are often given to glioma patients—but the drugs raise blood sugar, so they provide more fuel for glucose-hungry tumor cells.

The ketogenic diet was first used to treat malignant glioma in 1995,[12] and in the intervening years a number of rodent studies have indicated that the treatment is safe and effective. A smattering of human case reports of brain tumors that have shrunk or stopped growing are promising as well. In a study in China, researchers put eleven of thirty-four patients who had just undergone surgery for glioblastoma multiforme on a ketogenic diet in conjunction with chemotherapy and hyperbaric oxygen therapy; the survival time of the patients in the keto group was twice as long, on average, as that of patients who didn't change their diets.[13] Similarly, researchers at Harvard Medical School recently reviewed the studies on treating brain tumors with the keto diet and concluded that, while more research is needed, recognition of the benefits of this nontoxic remedy for malignant glioma might "pave the way for its establishment as an additional therapeutic pillar in neuro-oncological practice."[14]

Colon cancer

Colorectal cancer is the third most common cancer (excluding skin cancers) in both men and women in the United States, with a lifetime risk of one in twenty-two for men and one in twenty-four for women.[15] It's responsible for the deaths of more than fifty thousand people every year—and it appears that a carb- and sugar-rich diet increases the risk. In a study published in the *Journal of the National Cancer Institute,* researchers looked at carb consumption in nearly a thousand people with stage 3 colon cancer in which tumor cells had spread to the lymph nodes.[16] Those who consumed the most carbs and other foods that cause blood sugar to spike had an *80 percent* greater chance of dying from the disease or having a recurrence during the seven years of the study than those with the lowest carb consumption. The link was strongest in people who were overweight or obese.

The risk probably comes from insulin. In laboratory studies of colon cancer cells, insulin stimulates cell proliferation and inhibits their death. And in colon cancer patients, those with higher levels of C-peptide, a marker of long-term insulin production, had a significantly higher risk of dying than those with the lowest levels.

The ketogenic diet hasn't yet been studied in people with colon cancer, but a report in the journal *Nutrients* found that mice with colon cancer who were fed a ketogenic diet had significantly lower tumor weight and IL-6 levels (a measure of inflammation) than mice with the disease who were fed a standard carbohydrate diet.[17] Since the mice's tumor size shrunk as their blood levels of ketones rose, the researchers speculated that the anti-inflammatory effect of ketones might be responsible. A clinical trial in humans with advanced cancer of different types (breast, fallopian tube, lung, ovary, and colorectal) lends further credence to this idea. It found that blood ketone concentration was three times higher in patients whose cancer had stabilized or was in remission compared to those with disease progression.[18]

There's also evidence that keto-fed rodents are able to maintain their muscle mass and body weight better than rodents eating a carb-heavy diet — and maintaining weight during cancer treatment is vital, since losing weight and muscle mass is a potentially dangerous side effect of both the illness and conventional treatments.

Breast cancer

More than 266,000 women in the United States are diagnosed with invasive breast cancer every year, and another 64,000 are diagnosed with a noninvasive type.[19] Even more heartbreaking, breast cancer claims the lives of about 41,000 women in the United States every year.[20] But there are hopeful reports in the medical literature that the ketogenic diet could have a positive effect on the illness's trajectory. One paper shared the case of a woman who had just been diagnosed with a recurrence of HER2-positive cancer in her right breast who followed a strict ketogenic diet, along with high vitamin D supplementation, for three weeks before surgery.[21] HER2 is a growth-promoting protein on the outside of all breast cancer cells; when levels are higher than normal, they're called HER2 positive. Tumors that test positive for the protein tend to grow and spread faster than other types of breast cancer. When doctors analyzed her tumor after surgery, they discovered that it was no longer HER2 positive. In other words, the diet and vitamin D led to a significant change in a critical biomarker for breast cancer.

Similarly, a researcher at Boston College, along with a team from Turkey, reported on the case of a woman who had an aggressive type of breast cancer known as triple-negative.[22] She went on a ketogenic diet for six months, while undergoing regular chemotherapy and treatment with high heat and hyperbaric oxygen therapy. By the treatment's end, she was cured.

Studies with rodents are helping to explain why that might happen. In a paper published in *Cancer Research*, scientists found that mice fed meal that contained the amount of sugar found in the typical Western diet developed breast cancer tumors earlier, had larger tumors, and were more likely to have cancer that spread to their lungs than those on a low-sugar diet.[23] They also discovered that high dietary sugar triggers an inflammatory protein known as 12-LOX that increases the risk of breast cancer development and metastases.

Other research has shown that a higher intake of omega-3 fatty acids may protect women from developing breast tumors.[24] Losing weight can lower the risk as well[25] — particularly the excess fatty weight that collects deep in your belly, which the keto diet is specifically good at targeting. Taken together, the evidence provides hopeful clues that the keto diet could be an effective way to keep breast cells healthy — and play a meaningful, sometimes game-changing, role in treatment.

Prostate cancer

Interest is growing in using the ketogenic diet to treat the 165,000 men who are diagnosed with prostate cancer every year[26] — and maybe even prevent some of the 29,000 or so annual deaths that are attributed to the illness. In 2008, a team of scientists showed that mice on a no-carbohydrate ketogenic diet had significantly reduced tumor growth and prolonged survival compared to mice fed diets with either 72 percent carbs or 44 percent carbs.[27] Another study showed that mice on a no-carb diet lived longer than mice not on the diet;[28] more of their tumor cells died, and they had lower levels of inflammation and insulin as well.

It's virtually impossible for humans to follow a no-carb diet—but there's evidence that using a diet with up to 20 percent carbs produces similar results. A study in *Cancer Prevention Research* compared mice with prostate cancer that were fed no carbs, 10 percent carbs, and 20 percent carbs—and found they were equally effective in terms of the mice's survival.[29] At least one clinical trial in humans is currently under way. Researchers at the University of Maryland are trying to determine whether the ketogenic diet has a similar effect on men with the disease.

NINE POWERFUL AND PROVEN NATURAL CANCER STRATEGIES

Research in animals has also found signs that the keto diet might be helpful for those with lung, pancreatic, and gastric cancer—and could improve certain aspects of quality of life, including sleep and mood, in patients with advanced tumors that have spread to other locations in the body.[30] As important, the ketogenic diet is safe and free of dangerous side effects.

Based on my experience in treating cancer patients, I believe it's best to support ketosis with a number of other approaches that can magnify the diet's benefits and give sufferers the best shot at beating the disease. The following are natural strategies I recommended to my mom to strengthen and detoxify her body while she was battling cancer. I believe they worked in synergy with the diet to cure her of cancer. I recommend that you or your loved ones who are struggling with the disease try them, too.

Drink green juice. I had my mom pick up organic, locally grown produce at the farmers' market and make green juices every day with spinach, chard, celery, cucumber, cilantro, parsley, lime, ginger, and stevia. The combination can get rid of cancer-causing toxins that accumulate in your body—and the juice is jam-packed with antioxidants and other healing nutrients that can fortify your immune system's ability to fight disease.

Sprinkle on turmeric (curcumin) and other culinary herbs. A number of lab studies on cancer cells suggest that curcumin has anticancer effects. One paper showed that combining curcumin with chemotherapy reduced the number of bowel cancer cells better than chemotherapy alone.[31] Other herbs and spices, including cayenne, cinnamon, garlic, ginger, oregano, and rosemary, have powerful anticancer properties as well. Use them liberally when you cook.

Get more sunshine and vitamin D. A groundbreaking study published in the *American Journal of Clinical Nutrition* looked at twelve hundred postmenopausal women and found that after just one year of supplementing with vitamin D_3, the risk of developing cancer decreased by a whopping 77 percent.[32] Look for a daily supplement that contains 5,000 to 10,000 IU of vitamin D_3 and take it with foods containing coconut oil or a probiotic-rich drink like kefir to promote absorption. Optimize your D_3 supplements by getting twenty minutes of sun exposure every day.

Use frankincense and myrrh essential oils. These ancient oils have been shown to be effective for those with brain, breast, colon, pancreatic, prostate, and stomach cancer. Rub the two oils on your neck three times daily and drink 3 drops in 8 ounces of water three times every day as well.

Eat or supplement with reishi and cordyceps mushrooms. There's evidence these mushrooms can shrink tumors and bolster your immune system, as well as reduce chemotherapy-related nausea. If you're using a supplement, take the dose recommended on the bottle.

Up your antioxidant intake with superberries. The majority of fruit is too high in sugar for the ketogenic diet, but I encourage you to consume one serving of berries a day. Blueberries, cranberries, raspberries, and blackberries are some of the best and are packed with cancer-fighting antioxidants like flavanols, anthocyanins, and resveratrol. Also, organic exotic berry powders, like acai, camu camu, goji, maqui, and schisandra, are extremely high in antioxidants and are a great low-sugar, low-carb option. Just mix some into a glass of water, along with a pinch of stevia, for a refreshing drink.

Down bone broth. This healing elixir, made from the bones and innards of chicken, beef, lamb, or fish, is an excellent source of collagen, glycosaminoglycans, and other nutrients that help repair the lining of the gut—and a healthy gut environment can exponentially improve your overall health.

Choose probiotic foods and supplements. Speaking of your gut, it's vital to restore the health of its massive population of bacteria. Research shows that probiotic supplementation may help prevent tumor growth—a finding that makes sense since 80 percent of your immune system is located in your gut. Improving the health of your gut bacteria can also help you absorb more minerals—a capability that's especially important during chemo and will help you get every ounce of cancer-fighting nutrition you can out of my keto diet program. Supplement with 50 billion CFU once or twice a day.

Pray, meditate, or find other ways to relieve stress and promote positivity. It's difficult to quantify how important it is to maintain a positive outlook when you've been diagnosed with cancer, but I believe it's absolutely essential. Many of the lifestyle changes my mom began, including daily affirmations, prayer, walks in nature, and time with friends, were aimed at buoying her spirits and instilling a sense of peaceful calm—a feeling that's often tough to access when you're facing a frightening illness. Everyone has their favorite ways to do this. Whether it's yoga or laughter or nature walks or tai chi, find the activities that give you hope and happiness—and make them part of your daily routine. My favorite forms of meditation are prayer, gratitude, and reading the Bible. I see them as an essential part of my wellness strategy, as important as exercise or brushing my teeth. They lift my heart, give me hope, and keep me centered—and it's virtually impossible to overestimate how important those qualities can be. As it says in Proverbs 17:22, "A joyful heart is good medicine."

The ketogenic diet is the only dietary approach, aside from fasting, that can put your body into ketosis and, as a result, take aim at tumor cells' Achilles' heel: their reliance on glucose for fuel. Scientific evidence is rapidly affirming keto's remarkable potential to combat cancer on a molecular level by targeting its most glaring weakness. In many cases, it may be able to starve fledgling tumors and even stymie entrenched ones, offering those who are battling the disease an effective and forceful way to fight back. Moreover, committing to my keto diet program makes sense for everyone who is interested in cancer prevention. By putting your body into a fat-burning state, the program creates a protective environment in which this formidable foe is much less likely to gain a foothold and take root in the first place.

PART III

Your Personalized
Keto Plan

CHAPTER 11

The Keto Basic Plan

The Approach for Everyone Who Wants to Try Keto

Congratulations on choosing to go keto! I'm superexcited for the incredible results you're going to experience in the coming weeks. I designed this plan to be used for thirty days, but those who have more weight to lose or stubborn health conditions can extend it to sixty or ninety days. After that I recommend switching to the Forever Keto Cycling Plan, which is easier to maintain for the long term and provides a nice balance of healthy nutrients for your body, while still offering the benefits of ketosis. That said, it's important to start with full keto so your body reaps the advantages of being in ketosis for an extended, uninterrupted period of time. If you want some encouragement along the way, make sure to follow me on Facebook (Dr. Josh Axe) and Instagram @drjoshaxe. Share your results with me there. I'd love to help cheer you on!

PREPARING YOUR BODY FOR THE KETO DIET

Before you plunge into the diet, it's a good idea to do a brief transition phase of three to seven days. When you radically change your food intake and start loading up on superhealthy fat and minimizing your consumption of carbs, it takes your body at least a few days to adjust. A high-fat diet is more demanding on the liver and gallbladder, for instance, and eating fewer carbs means your blood sugar can drop. This run-up period is designed to help your body acclimate to those changes, so once you're on the diet you're prepped and ready to experience its full benefits.

Here's what I want you to do during the preparation phase:

Gradually increase your intake of healthy fat. Start adding avocado to your eggs and your salads, use coconut oil and almond milk and coconut milk in your smoothies, and eat a handful of nuts in place of your usual snack.

Start paying attention to carbs. You don't necessarily need to cut back just yet, but notice where your carbs are coming from and begin purging your pantry and fridge of the carb- and sugar-heavy foods you won't be eating once you begin the thirty-day plan. If it's not in the house, you're much less likely to indulge.

Consume plenty of water. It cleanses your body and is good for you no matter what diet you're on. But it's especially important as you're preparing for keto, since many people lose water weight in the beginning of the program due to the diet's low sugar and lower sodium content. (Both sugar and sodium cause your body to hold on to water.) Aim to drink at least half your body weight in ounces. In other words, if you weigh 150 pounds, drink *at least* 75 ounces every day.

HERE WE GO: KETO!

Now that you've set the stage, you're ready to start the diet itself. The most important aspect of the keto diet is your macros. You should consume 75 percent fat, 20 percent protein, and 5 percent carbs. It might help to visualize a plate with those proportions. But don't worry about doing tons of math to make sure you're eating the right quantities of each macronutrient. On page 171 I've laid out an entire thirty-day meal plan to make it supereasy. You can also utilize any of the more than eighty wholesome, delicious, simple recipes in Chapter 17. Each one contains the ideal proportions of fat, protein, and carbs, so you don't have to sweat the details. All of the recipes are in regular rotation in our home. I think you'll love them as much as Chelsea and I do.

I explained the keto flu in Chapter 3, but as a reminder, here are sev-

YOUR KETO PLATE

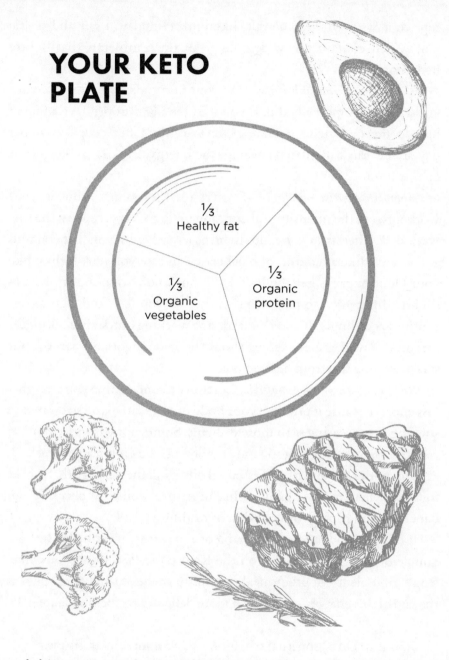

eral things you can do to minimize the likelihood of suffering symptoms and transition seamlessly into ketosis:

Continue drinking plenty of water.

Sprinkle a little sea salt on your food. When you cut out packaged and prepared foods, you're going to consume less sodium. It's a good idea to replace it with wholesome salt, like pink Himalayan salt and Celtic salt, which contain the widest range of trace minerals that bolster hydration.

Consume caffeinated beverages. As your body adjusts to ketosis, your energy may temporarily dip. If you start feeling droopy, have a cup of black coffee or matcha green tea. Don't overdo it, but a cup or two per day of a healthy caffeinated beverage (no energy drinks!) can keep your energy high.

Approach exercise mindfully. If you're used to going all out in your workouts, cut the intensity and duration by 10 to 20 percent for the first week of the diet. It's a good idea to bring a snack with you that contains a few carbs, like a handful of blueberries, in case you start feeling like your blood sugar is getting low. Everyone's body responds to ketosis slightly differently, so pay attention to how you feel, and adjust your routine accordingly. If you're not used to working out, start walking 20 minutes a day. Regular exercise should be a nonnegotiable part of your stay-well program from here on out.

Reduce stress as much as possible. Cortisol can undermine your weight-loss efforts because it prompts your body to store fat—and stress makes sticking to any eating plan more difficult. Some of my favorite tension reducers are listening to good music, praying, and taking a healing bath at night with Epsom salts and essential oils. Find the strategy that works for you, whether it's yoga, walking in nature, doing tai chi, singing, dancing, doing crossword puzzles, or reading a novel.

It can be difficult to get the hang of a new way of eating, so here's a sample of what a typical day on the Keto Basic Plan might look like. You'll find plenty of other meal options in the seven-day meal plan at the end of this chapter—and even more delicious recipes in Chapter 17.

> 7:30 a.m. Do a "spiritual triathlon": five minutes of gratitude practice, five minutes of reading the Bible or a book about personal growth, five minutes of prayer or meditation.
>
> 8:00 a.m. Drink a keto smoothie with coconut milk, keto protein or collagen protein (vanilla is a tasty option for smoothies), and almond butter. Take exogenous ketones, a multivitamin, and

digestive enzymes. If you have digestive issues, take a probiotic as well.

9:00 a.m. Have a glass of matcha green tea or coffee with MCT oil and/or ghee.

12:00 p.m. Enjoy a grass-fed burger lettuce wrap with spinach salad and avocado. Take digestive enzymes.

5:00 p.m. Exercise for 20-plus minutes. Weight training, HIIT training, cardio, and yoga all work for exercise. If you're unable to exercise, take a walk.

6:30 p.m. Consume a keto-friendly dinner. See the recipes in Chapter 17 for ideas. Take digestive enzymes.

9:00 p.m. Turn off technology! Do something relaxing to prepare your brain for sleep: Read a book, write in your gratitude journal, take a warm bath with jasmine oil, meditate, or pray.

10:30 p.m. Lights out.

THE TOP FOUR SUPPLEMENTS TO SUPPORT THE KETO BASIC PLAN

As I explained in Chapter 5, a variety of supplements can support your efforts to get into ketosis and ensure that you maximize the effects of the plan. Now is the time to revisit that chapter and see which ones make the most sense for your particular health issues. In general, here are the top four I recommend to everyone who is doing the Keto Basic Plan.

1. **Exogenous ketones.** Exogenous ketones will help you get into ketosis more quickly. They can be enormously beneficial, especially during the first week or two on the program. If you have a powdered form, take 6 grams once or twice a day, with the first dose in the morning. If you have capsules, which are usually combined with synergistic ingredients, take 2 grams.

2. **Keto protein or keto collagen.** Choose keto protein if you struggle to consume enough protein in your diet and you're interested in muscle building. Opt for keto collagen if one of your top concerns is

healthy aging and protecting your joints, hair, skin, and nails. For keto protein, each serving should contain 10 to 15 grams of protein and 10 to 15 grams of fat from bone broth, which offers a superhealthy source of both protein and fat as well as medium–chain triglycerides, perhaps the healthiest fat available. For keto collagen, look for one that has at least 3 grams of fat per serving. Because these products are optimized for ketosis, they help flip the switch from carb burning to fat burning and provide sustained energy. Take 1 or 2 scoops daily with a glass of water or coffee or your morning smoothie.

YOUR KETOGENIC DIET MEALS

AT A GLANCE

For best results, follow this caloric breakout:

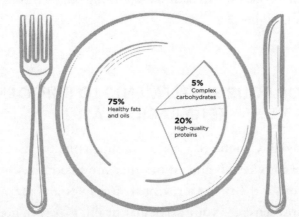

5%
Complex carbohydrates

75%
Healthy fats and oils

20%
High-quality proteins

SAMPLE CHOICES INCLUDE:

HEALTHY FATS AND OILS	FATS		OILS
	Avocados	Coconut milk	Avocado oil
	Ghee	Nuts	Chia seed oil
	Grass-fed butter	Olives	Coconut oil
	Almond butter	Seeds (flax, chia and hemp)	Extra virgin olive oil
	Cacao	Tahini	Flaxseed oil
			Macadamia nut oil
			Sesame oil
HIGH-QUALITY PROTEINS	Wild-caught fish	Bone broth	Grass-fed bison
	Grass-fed beef	Chicken	Lamb
	Eggs (chicken and duck)	Collagen protein	Turkey
		Cottage cheese	Turkey bacon
	Bone broth protein	Duck	Venison
VEGETABLES AND FRUITS	Artichokes	Cauliflower	Onions
	Asparagus	Garlic	Romaine lettuce
	Berries	Green beans	Spinach
	Broccoli	Kale	Squash/Zucchini
	Brussels sprouts	Lemons and limes	
	Cabbage	Mushrooms	

3. **A keto-friendly digestive enzymes supplement** with soil-based microorganisms to help you break down fat and promote the growth of healthy bacteria in your gut. Take the dosage recommended on the bottle with meals one to three times daily.

4. **A multivitamin** that contains all the nutrients you might be missing, now that you've given up some healthy veggies and fruits for the initial thirty days. My keto diet plan's high fat content allows you to fully absorb fat-soluble vitamins, like A, D, E, and K, so choose a multi with healthy quantities of those nutrients in particular. Also, opt for one that contains several times more than the recommended value of B vitamins, particularly B_{12}, since you won't be getting as much through your diet—and B vitamins are critical for maintaining your daily energy levels. Since formulations vary, take the standard dosage recommended on the bottle.

SAMPLE THIRTY-DAY MEAL PLAN

THE KETO BASIC MEAL PLAN

Day 1

Breakfast
> Keto scrambled eggs (3 eggs, spinach, mushrooms, cherry tomatoes, and seasonings to taste and cooked in coconut oil)
> *Turmeric Golden Milk* (page 244)

Lunch
> *Lamb Burger* (page 261)
> Side salad

Snack (optional)
> ½ cup of blackberries served with 1 tablespoon of almond butter

Dinner
> 6 ounces of wild-caught salmon cooked in 2 tablespoons of coconut oil

6 ounces of steamed Brussels sprouts topped with 1 tablespoon of flax oil and seasoned to taste

Day 2

Breakfast

Vanilla Bean Smoothie (page 241)

Lunch

Zucchini noodles topped with cherry tomatoes and avocado sauce (avocado, lemon juice, pine nuts, water, and seasonings to taste)
Side salad

Snack (optional)

1 slice *Keto Bread* (page 280)

Dinner

6 ounces of organic, grass-fed bison cooked in 2 tablespoons of coconut oil
6 ounces of green beans sautéed in 1 to 2 tablespoons of ghee

Dessert

Keto Fudgesicle (page 293)

Day 3

Breakfast

Keto Pancakes (page 236)
Turkey Breakfast Sausage (page 237)
Keto Coffee (page 244)

Lunch

Chicken Salad Lettuce Wraps (page 245)
½ avocado

Snack (optional)

½ cup of goat's milk cottage cheese with a handful of berries

Dinner

6 ounces of organic, grass-fed lamb cooked in 2 tablespoons of coconut oil

5 ounces of steamed cabbage topped with 1 tablespoon of olive oil and seasoned to taste

---
Day 4

Breakfast

Yogurt parfait (*Granola* [page 283], unsweetened coconut yogurt, fresh berries, unsweetened shredded coconut, almond butter, and cacao nibs)

Matcha green tea

Lunch

Strawberry Spinach Salad with Poppy Seed Dressing (page 270)

Snack (optional)

½ avocado

Dinner

6 ounces of organic, free-range chicken cooked in 2 tablespoons of coconut oil

Cajun Collard Greens (page 273)

Dessert

½ cup of strawberries dipped in 2 ounces of dark chocolate

Day 5

Breakfast

Low-Carb Egg Muffin (page 237)

Lunch

Steak fajitas (6 ounces of steak, red and green pepper, onion, olive oil, and lemon juice) served in romaine lettuce boats

6 ounces of summer squash sautéed in 1 to 2 tablespoons of ghee

Snack (optional)

½ cup of raspberries served with 1 tablespoon of almond butter

Dinner

Coconut Chicken Tenders (page 258)

Steamed broccoli and cauliflower drizzled with 2 tablespoons of
tahini and sea salt

Day 6

Breakfast

Keto Cashew Cookie Shake (page 242)

Lunch

6 ounces of wild-caught halibut cooked in 2 tablespoons of
coconut oil

9 ounces of celery sautéed in 2 tablespoons of flax oil

½ cup of strawberries

Snack (optional)

Keto Cookie Dough Bar (page 281)

Dinner

Vegetarian Ceviche with Mushrooms (page 259)

5 ounces of sliced cucumber drizzled with lemon juice and olive
oil and seasoned to taste

Dessert

Lemon Bar (page 286)

Day 7

Breakfast

3 eggs fried in 1 to 2 tablespoons of avocado oil

Sautéed kale

Keto Coffee (page 244)

Lunch
> 4 to 6 ounces of tuna salad (wild-caught canned tuna with 2 to 3 tablespoons of avocado mayo) served over a bed of mixed greens
> ½ cup of blueberries

Snack (optional)
> Celery sticks served with *Cinnamon Nut Butter* (page 276)

Dinner
> *Keto Buffalo Chicken Wings* (page 256)
> 6 ounces of steamed Brussels sprouts topped with 1 tablespoon of flax oil and seasoned to taste

---
Day 8

Breakfast
> *Keto Green Smoothie* (page 243)

Lunch
> 6 ounces of organic, grass-fed beef cooked in 2 tablespoons of coconut oil
> 9 ounces of grilled asparagus drizzled with 1 to 2 tablespoons of olive oil and seasoned to taste
> ½ avocado

Snack (optional)
> *Keto Fat Bomb* (page 279)

Dinner
> Burrito bowl (cauliflower rice, black beans, bell peppers, avocado, red onion, and chicken or beef, topped with olive oil and lime juice)

Day 9

Breakfast
> *Chia Pudding* (page 279)

Lunch

Steak fajitas (6 ounces of steak, red and green pepper, onion, olive oil, and lemon juice) served in romaine lettuce boats

6 ounces of summer squash sautéed in 1 to 2 tablespoons of ghee

Snack (optional)

½ cup of blueberries and 1 ounce of hard cheese, cubed

Dinner

Lamb Burger (page 261)

Cheesy Broccoli (page 267)

Dessert

½ cup of raspberries dipped in 2 ounces of dark chocolate

Day 10

Breakfast

Veggie Omelet (page 239)

Turkey Breakfast Sausage (page 237)

Lunch

6 ounces of organic, free-range turkey cooked in 2 tablespoons of sesame oil

5 ounces of steamed spinach topped with 1 tablespoon of olive oil and seasoned to taste

Snack (optional)

Celery sticks served with Cinnamon Nut Butter (page 276)

Dinner

Salmon Cakes with Garlic Aioli (page 255)

6 ounces of green beans sautéed in 1 to 2 tablespoons of ghee

---

Day 11

Breakfast

Keto Pancakes (page 236)

Lunch

Leftover *Salmon Cakes with Garlic Aioli* (page 255)

6 ounces of zucchini sautéed in 1 to 2 tablespoons of coconut oil

½ cup of blueberries

Snack (optional)

½ avocado (optional)

Dinner

Slow Cooker Beef and Broccoli (page 263)

Cauliflower Rice with Cilantro and Lime (page 268)

Side salad

Dessert

Keto Peanut Butter Cookie (page 287)

Day 12

Breakfast

Yogurt parfait (leftover *Granola* [page 283], unsweetened coconut
yogurt, fresh berries, unsweetened shredded coconut, almond
butter, and cacao nibs)

Matcha green tea

Lunch

Coconut Chicken Tenders (page 258)

5 ounces of steamed spinach topped with 1 tablespoon of olive oil
and seasoned to taste

½ avocado

Snack (optional)

Celery sticks served with *Cinnamon Nut Butter* (page 276)

Dinner

6 ounces of organic, grass-fed lamb cooked in 2 tablespoons of
coconut oil

6 ounces of green beans sautéed in 1 to 2 tablespoons of ghee

Day 13

Breakfast

Blueberry Smoothie (page 240)

Lunch

Leftover *Slow Cooker Beef and Broccoli* (page 263)

Side salad

Snack (optional)

Collagen-Boosting Blueberry Muffin (page 282)

Dinner

Raw walnut tacos (raw walnuts, coconut aminos,
  seasonings to taste, and romaine lettuce leaves) served
  with guacamole

5 ounces of sliced cucumber drizzled with lemon juice and olive
  oil and seasoned to taste

Dessert

Chocolate Avocado Mousse (page 285)

Day 14

Breakfast

Grain-Free Quiche (page 238)

Turmeric Golden Milk (page 244)

Lunch

Cauliflower Steak (page 261)

6 ounces of summer squash sautéed in 1 to 2 tablespoons of ghee

Snack (optional)

Chia Pudding (page 279)

Dinner

Chicken Pesto (page 256)

9 ounces of grilled asparagus drizzled with 1 to 2 tablespoons of
  olive oil and seasoned to taste

Day 15

Breakfast

Keto Collagen Shake (page 240)

Lunch

Leftover *Chicken Pesto* (page 256)

5 ounces of steamed kale topped with 1 to 2 tablespoons of olive oil and seasoned to taste

½ cup strawberries and 1 ounce of hard cheese

Snack (optional)

Keto Deviled Eggs (page 284)

Dinner

Zucchini Lasagna (page 264)

Side salad

Day 16

Breakfast

Keto Chocolate Smoothie (page 242)

Lunch

Buffalo Chili (page 252)

Side salad

Snack (optional)

½ cup of goat's milk cottage cheese with a handful of berries

Dinner

6 ounces of organic, free-range chicken baked in 2 tablespoons of butter and seasoned with Italian seasoning

6 ounces of green beans sautéed in 1 to 2 tablespoons of ghee

Dessert

Keto Chocolate Chip Cookie (page 288)

Day 17

Breakfast

Turmeric Smoothie (page 241)

Lunch

Leftover *Buffalo Chili* (page 252)
Side salad
½ cup of blackberries

Snack (optional)

Keto Cookie Dough Bar (page 281)

Dinner

6 ounces of organic, free-range turkey cooked in 2 tablespoons of coconut oil
Cajun Collard Greens (page 273)

Day 18

Breakfast

3 eggs fried in 1 to 2 tablespoons of avocado oil
Turkey Breakfast Sausage (page 237)
Sautéed kale
Matcha green tea

Lunch

Burrito bowl (cauliflower rice, black beans, bell peppers, avocado, red onion, and chicken or beef, topped with olive oil and lime juice)

Snack (optional)

Keto Fat Bombs (page 279)

Dinner

Cauliflower Steak (page 261)
9 ounces of asparagus drizzled with 1 to 2 tablespoons of olive oil and seasoned to taste

Dessert
> *Keto Cheesecake* (page 291)

Day 19

Breakfast
> *Grain-Free Quiche* (page 238)
> *Keto Coffee* (page 244)

Lunch
> Steak fajitas (6 ounces of steak, red and green pepper, onion, olive
> oil, and lemon juice) served in romaine lettuce boats
> 6 ounces of summer squash sautéed in 1 to 2 tablespoons of ghee

Snack (optional)
> *Kale Chips* (page 281)

Dinner
> 6 ounces of organic, free-range turkey cooked in 2 tablespoons of
> coconut oil
> 9 ounces of grilled asparagus drizzled with 1 to 2 tablespoons of
> olive oil and seasoned to taste

Day 20

Breakfast
> *Vanilla Bean Smoothie* (page 241)

Lunch
> Zucchini noodles topped with cherry tomatoes and avocado sauce
> (avocado, lemon juice, pine nuts, water, and seasonings to taste)
> Side salad

Snack (optional)
> Celery sticks served with *Cinnamon Nut Butter* (page 276)

Dinner
> *Steak and Veggie Kebabs* (page 254)
> *Strawberry Spinach Salad with Poppy Seed Dressing* (page 270)

Dessert
   Peppermint Patty (page 285)

Day 21

Breakfast
   Keto Pancakes (page 236)
   3 slices of turkey bacon
   Matcha green tea

Lunch
   Raw walnut tacos (raw walnuts, coconut aminos, seasonings to
      taste, and romaine lettuce leaves) served with guacamole
   5 ounces of sliced cucumber drizzled with lemon juice and olive
      oil and seasoned to taste

Snack (optional)
   ½ cup of goat's milk cottage cheese with a handful of berries

Dinner
   Chicken Vegetable Soup (page 250)
   Salad of romaine lettuce, turkey bacon bits, and tomato served
      with *Cashew Caesar Dressing* (page 275)

Day 22

Breakfast
   Low-Carb Egg Muffin (page 237)
   Turmeric Golden Milk (page 244)

Lunch
   Leftover *Chicken Vegetable Soup* (page 250)
   Side salad
   ½ cup of raspberries

Snack (optional)
   Chia Pudding (page 279)

Dinner

> *Zucchini Lasagna* (page 264)
>
> Salad of romaine lettuce, turkey bacon bits, and tomato served
> with *Cashew Caesar Dressing* (page 275)

Day 23

Breakfast

> *Keto Cashew Cookie Shake* (page 242)

Lunch

> *Chicken Pesto* (page 256)
>
> *Grilled Asparagus* (page 271)

Snack (optional)

> ½ cup of blueberries served with 1 tablespoon of almond butter

Dinner

> 6 ounces of organic, grass-fed beef cooked in 2 tablespoons of
> coconut oil
>
> 5 ounces of sliced cucumber drizzled with lemon juice and olive
> oil and seasoned to taste

Dessert

> ½ cup of strawberries dipped in 2 ounces of dark chocolate

Day 24

Breakfast

> *Grain-Free Quiche* (page 238)

Lunch

> Steak fajitas (6 ounces of steak, red and green pepper, onion, olive
> oil, and lemon juice) served in romaine lettuce boats
>
> 6 ounces of summer squash sautéed in 1 to 2 tablespoons of ghee

Snack (optional)

> 1 slice *Keto Bread* (page 280)

Dinner

    Thai Coconut Chicken Soup (page 260)

    Side salad

Day 25

Breakfast

    Blueberry Smoothie (page 240)

Lunch

    Egg Tahini Salad (page 248)

Snack (optional)

    Celery sticks served with *Cinnamon Nut Butter* (page 276)

Dinner

    6 ounces of organic, free-range chicken baked in 2 tablespoons of
        butter and seasoned with Italian seasoning

    6 ounces of green beans sautéed in 1 to 2 tablespoons of ghee

Dessert

    Toasted Coconut Macaroons (page 289)

Day 26

Breakfast

    Low-Carb Egg Muffin (page 237)

Lunch

    Chicken Salad Lettuce Wraps (page 245)

    ½ cup of raspberries

Snack (optional)

    Granola (page 283) served with ½ cup of mixed berries

Dinner

    Spaghetti and Marinara Meat Sauce (page 253)

    9 ounces of grilled asparagus drizzled with 1 to 2 tablespoons of
        olive oil and seasoned to taste

Day 27

Breakfast

Keto Chocolate Smoothie (page 242)

Lunch

BLT Turkey Wrap (page 246)
Sliced bell pepper
½ cup of blackberries

Snack (optional)

½ cup of goat's milk cottage cheese with a handful of berries

Dinner

Zucchini noodles topped with cherry tomatoes and avocado sauce
(avocado, lemon juice, pine nuts, water, and seasonings to taste)
Side salad

Dessert

Keto Brownie (page 290)

Day 28

Breakfast

3 eggs fried in 1 to 2 tablespoons of avocado oil
3 slices of turkey bacon
Sautéed kale

Lunch

Avocado stuffed with diced tomatoes, cucumbers, bell peppers,
onion and Tahini Lemon Dressing (page 275)
Side salad
½ cup of strawberries

Snack (optional)

Celery sticks served with Cinnamon Nut Butter (page 276)

Dinner

    6 ounces of organic, free-range turkey cooked in 2 tablespoons of coconut oil

    9 ounces of grilled asparagus drizzled with 1 to 2 tablespoons of olive oil and seasoned to taste

---

Day 29

Breakfast

    Probiotic Kefir Smoothie (page 243)

Lunch

    6 ounces of organic, grass-fed beef cooked in 2 tablespoons of coconut oil

    5 ounces of sliced cucumber drizzled with lemon juice and olive oil and seasoned to taste

Snack (optional)

    ½ cup of blueberries served with 1 tablespoon of almond butter

Dinner

    Keto Florentine Pizza (page 265)

    Side salad

Dessert

    Keto Brownie (page 290)

Day 30

Breakfast

    Yogurt parfait (leftover *Granola* [page 283], unsweetened coconut yogurt, fresh berries, unsweetened shredded coconut, almond butter, and cacao nibs)

    Matcha green tea

Lunch

Zucchini noodles topped with cherry tomatoes and avocado sauce
(avocado, lemon juice, pine nuts, water, and seasonings to
taste)

Side salad

Snack (optional)

½ cup of goat's milk cottage cheese with a handful of berries

Dinner

Keto Beef Tacos in Romaine Boats (page 246)

Side salad

CHAPTER 12

The Keto Fasting Plan

Using Intermittent Fasting to Bolster Keto and Restore Your Health

Food is medicine. The nutrients you consume give your cells the building blocks they need to repair, rejuvenate, and function normally. But food doesn't heal the body. *The body heals itself.* As you already know by now, a wholesome ketogenic diet, which reduces blood glucose and insulin and contains plenty of healthy fat to enhance nutrient absorption, is one of the best ways to set the stage for healing because it puts your body into ketosis. Another powerful tool is fasting. Just as your cells fix glitches and replicate while you sleep, they also undergo critical renewal and restoration when you're not eating.

When you go without food for more than 12 hours, your digestive system gets a chance to rest, and within 12 to 36 hours your body enters ketosis and starts burning fat for fuel, according to a 2018 paper in *Obesity*,[1] the same healthy metabolic state you reach with my keto diet program, allowing you to double down on its fat-burning benefits. The paper's team of researchers, including Mark Mattson, PhD, chief of the Laboratory of Neurosciences at the National Institute on Aging Intramural Research Program, concluded that even relatively short periods of repeated fasting, known as intermittent fasting (IF), trigger this metabolic switch from glucose burning to fat burning and, as a result, have the potential to reduce fat and preserve muscle mass in people who are over-weight. Moreover, they say, IF regimens activate molecular signaling pathways that "optimize physiological function, enhance performance, and slow aging and disease processes."

Whether you fast or not, you're going to be in ketosis when you follow my keto diet program. But combining my keto diet plan and intermittent fasting is helpful for anyone who wants to accelerate fat loss, struggles with overeating, has reached a weight-loss plateau, or wants to protect themselves from cancer and neurological disorders and other diseases of aging.

I've found that a form of intermittent fasting known as "time-restricted eating"—in which you consume all your meals within a six-, eight-, or ten-hour window every day and fast for the other eighteen, sixteen, or fourteen hours—works particularly well with my keto diet program because it dovetails with the way our ancient ancestors ate, when people lived by rhythms dictated by the rising and setting of the sun.

Our bodies are still designed for daily fasts of at least twelve hours, but in our 24/7 culture, it's rare for people to stay within that eating window. A study in the journal *Cell Metabolism* found that more than half of adults eat for fifteen hours or longer every day.[2] The study also found that when overweight participants who typically ate for more than fourteen hours a day restricted their food intake to a ten- to eleven-hour window, they lost weight and reported that they felt more energetic and were sleeping more soundly—results that they maintained during a year of follow-up. Animal studies of time-restricted feeding have shown that the approach can bolster overall health, too.[3] And I've noticed vast improvements in patients' digestion when they restrict their food-consumption window.

The benefits of adding intermittent fasting come from enhancing and deepening your experience of ketosis—as well as from allowing your system to rest, which supports regeneration and cleansing. Think of it this way: If you have a cut on your arm and pick at it every hour, it won't ever heal. The same thing happens when you don't give your

NUTRIENT TIMING AT A GLANCE

For an 8-hour eating window:

12:00 a.m.   12:00 p.m.   12:00 a.m.

Lunch	12:00 p.m. to 1:00 p.m.
Snack (optional)	3:30 p.m. to 4:00 p.m.
Dinner	7:00 p.m. to 8:00 p.m.

For a 6-hour eating window:

12:00 a.m.   12:00 p.m.   12:00 a.m.

Lunch	1:00 p.m. to 2:00 p.m.
Snack (optional)	3:30 p.m. to 4:00 p.m.
Dinner	6:00 p.m. to 7:00 p.m.

For a 4-hour eating window:

12:00 a.m.   12:00 p.m.   12:00 a.m.

Lunch	2:00 p.m. to 3:00 p.m.
Snack (optional)	3:30 p.m. to 4:00 p.m.
Dinner	5:00 p.m. to 6:00 p.m.

cells enough time to undergo daily restoration. Without a pause in eating and digestion, your body doesn't have adequate time to address the underlying abnormalities that accrue with daily wear and tear.

Adding intermittent fasting to my keto diet will take your regimen up a notch—but it adds another level of commitment and intensity. As a result, I recommend it for those who are familiar with ketosis and who have been on a ketogenic diet for a week or two and have adjusted to burning fat for fuel.

HOW TO PAIR INTERMITTENT FASTING WITH KETO

To take advantage of intermittent fasting while on my keto diet, pick an eating window that will work for you most of the time—but don't let perfection be the enemy of the good. Experiment and find what fits best with your lifestyle. Some people like to eat from 10:00 a.m. or 12:00 p.m. to 6:00 p.m. Others prefer to shift their window earlier or later. If you start with a six-hour window and find it's too restrictive, lengthen it by an hour or two and see if that works better. You also might want to ease into the approach by simply skipping a meal, like breakfast. When I practice keto fasting, I typically have matcha green tea or coffee in the morning, eat my first meal at 12:00 p.m., have a snack at 3:00 p.m., and eat dinner at 6:00 p.m. It's easy and makes me feel great.

If you exercise (and I recommend that you do), you'll get the biggest fat burn if you do so in a fasted state, so lots of people like to work out in the morning before they've eaten. Regardless of when you exercise, have your biggest meal after your workout so you can replenish the calories you need to fuel your body and prevent a drop in energy and focus.

You can have water or black coffee or tea when you first wake up and remain in a fasting state. During your eating window, consume the healthy, keto-optimized recipes in Chapter 17. Don't worry about calories. Just eat when you're hungry and stop when you're full—and enjoy the benefits of a deeper keto experience.

To help you get started, here's an example of what a typical day might look like. You might want to have a more extended eating window when you're first trying time-restricted eating—maybe you have your first meal at 10:30 a.m. or 11:00 a.m. but gradually shrink the window so you wind up with a day that looks something like this:

7:30 a.m. Do a "spiritual triathlon": five minutes of gratitude practice, five minutes of reading the Bible or a book about personal growth, five minutes of prayer or meditation.

8:00 a.m. Drink a cup of plain matcha green tea or coffee. If you're hungry throughout the morning, have decaffeinated, calorie-free tea, coffee, or water.

11:30 a.m. Go for a 20-minute walk.

12:00 p.m. Have a hearty keto lunch. (See the sample seven-day meal plan at the end of this chapter.) Take probiotics and herb supplements.

3:00 p.m. Drink a glass of vegetable juice with a scoop of keto protein and keto collagen.

5:00 or 6:00 p.m. Go for a 30-minute walk or do yoga, hit the gym, or go for a run or bike ride. If you're used to exercising more, you can go for up to 60 minutes, but don't push it as your body adjusts to fasting.

6:00 or 7:00 p.m. Consume a healthy, keto-friendly dinner and a probiotic.

9:00 p.m. Turn off technology! Do something relaxing to prepare your brain for sleep: Read a book, write in your gratitude journal, take a warm bath with jasmine oil, meditate, or pray.

10:30 p.m. Lights out.

THE TOP FOUR SUPPLEMENTS TO SUPPORT YOUR KETO FASTING PLAN

1. **Keto protein** will give you a stable, perfectly balanced source of fat and protein to ensure you feel full and help you restrict your eating to your chosen window of time. Add a scoop to your midday smoothie or green juice.

2. **Keto collagen** is a good addition as well because it supports the health of your skin, hair, joints, and gut. Add a scoop to water or your morning tea or coffee to boost your overall intake of collagen.

3. **Probiotics** will support fasting's healthy effects on your digestion and microbiome. Look for a probiotic supplement that contains soil-based microorganisms, like *Saccharomyces boulardii*, *Bacillus clausii*, *Bacillus coagulans*, and *Bacillus subtilis*. It will help you adapt to a keto

lifestyle and promote digestive healing. Take 50 billion CFU one or two times a day.

4. **Herbs** like cinnamon, turmeric, holy basil, and ashwagandha support healthy blood sugar levels. Consuming them will promote and intensify the healing effect of fasting. These supplement formulations vary, so follow the standard dosage on the bottle.

SAMPLE SEVEN-DAY MEAL PLAN

Day 1

Morning
> *Keto Coffee* (page 244)

Lunch
> 6-ounce grilled chicken breast in a lettuce wrap
> 9 ounces of asparagus drizzled with 1 to 2 tablespoons of olive oil and seasoned to taste
> ½ avocado

Snack (optional)
> 1 slice *Keto Bread* (page 280)

Dinner
> *Steak and Veggie Kebabs* (page 254)
> Side salad

Day 2

Morning
> Matcha green tea

Lunch
> *BLT Turkey Wrap* (page 246)
> Sliced bell peppers dipped in hummus

Snack (optional)
> *Keto Cookie Dough Bar* (page 281)

Dinner

>   6 ounces of organic, grass-fed bison cooked in 2 tablespoons of coconut oil
>
>   5 ounces of sliced cucumber drizzled with lemon juice and olive oil and seasoned to taste
>
>   *Cauliflower Rice with Cilantro and Lime* (page 268)

Day 3

Morning

>   *Keto Coffee* (page 244)

Lunch

>   *Vegetarian Ceviche with Mushrooms* (page 259)
>   Side salad

Snack (optional)

>   ½ cup of raspberries served with 1 tablespoon of almond butter

Dinner

>   6 ounces of organic, grass-fed lamb cooked in 2 tablespoons of coconut oil
>
>   6 ounces of zucchini sautéed in 1 to 2 tablespoons of coconut oil

Day 4

Morning

>   Matcha green tea

Lunch

>   *Strawberry Spinach Salad with Poppy Seed Dressing* (page 270)

Snack (optional)

>   ½ avocado

Dinner

>   6 ounces of organic, free-range chicken cooked in 2 tablespoons of coconut oil

5 ounces of steamed kale topped with 1 to 2 tablespoons of olive oil
and seasoned to taste

¼ cup of blueberries

Day 5

Morning

Keto Coffee (page 244)

Lunch

Leftover organic, free-range chicken

5 ounces of steamed spinach topped with 1 tablespoon of olive oil
and seasoned to taste

½ avocado

Snack (optional)

½ cup of blackberries served with 1 tablespoon of almond butter

Dinner

Spaghetti and Marinara Meat Sauce (page 253)
Side salad

Day 6

Morning

Matcha green tea

Lunch

Egg Tahini Salad (page 248)
½ cup of strawberries

Snack (optional)

Keto Fat Bomb (page 279)

Dinner

6 ounces of wild-caught salmon cooked in 2 tablespoons of
coconut oil

6 ounces of green beans sautéed in 1 to 2 tablespoons of ghee

Day 7

Morning

Keto Coffee (page 244)

Lunch

6 ounces of organic, free-range chicken cooked in 2 tablespoons of
coconut oil

6 ounces of summer squash sautéed in 1 to 2 tablespoons of ghee

Snack (optional)

½ cup of blueberries with 1 tablespoon of almond butter

Dinner

Slow Cooker Beef and Broccoli (page 263)

9 ounces of grilled asparagus drizzled with 1 to 2 tablespoons of
olive oil and seasoned to taste

CHAPTER 13

The Keto Vegan Plan

How to Make Keto Fit Your Lifestyle

I had just finished a yoga class one day when the twenty-nine-year-old instructor, Claire, approached me. Her face looked sunken and sallow and her eyes had dark circles beneath them. She told me she was vegan and she'd been trying to go keto while staying away from meat. She said she felt bloated, her joints ached, and she was tired all the time. In Chinese medicine, she had what's known as a kidney qi deficiency. From a functional medicine perspective, it's similar to adrenal fatigue and can lead to hypothyroidism.

I explained that she probably had a collagen deficiency and wasn't getting enough vitamin B_{12}. I suggested she supplement her vegan approach to keto with a keto-optimized collagen, along with probiotics, B_{12}, and ashwagandha to balance her stress hormone, cortisol. I acknowledged that collagen isn't vegan. "But I believe you'll find that it will make a remarkable difference," I said.

When I saw her two weeks later, the change was dramatic. Her skin was glowing, her joint pain had gone away, and her energy had returned. She said, "I haven't had meat or animal products in eight years. I can't believe one scoop of collagen a day, plus a few supplements, was all it took to make me feel well. I literally feel and look like a different person."

Six percent of Americans now identify as vegan. If you're one of them, I admire your commitment to the planet, animal welfare, and your own health. As a functional medicine doctor, I also know that avoiding meat products can put you at risk for certain deficiencies, particularly B$_{12}$ and collagen—and it's not the best approach if you've been diagnosed with type 2 diabetes or you're overweight, conditions for which my keto diet is ideal. Here's the good news: You can absolutely do a vegan version of my keto diet program.

THE VEGAN APPROACH TO KETO

In order to make keto vegan-friendly, you'll need to consume lots of low-carb vegetables, like asparagus, avocado, broccoli, cauliflower, kale, mushrooms, spinach, and zucchini. Since you'll need to get 75 percent of your calories from fat, you'll also need to load up on healthy plant-based sources, like coconut oil, MCT oil, extra-virgin olive oil, avocado, avocado oil, coconut butter, macadamia nut oil, walnut oil, vegan cheeses, vegan butter, coconut- or nut-based yogurt, and nuts and seeds. Get plenty of fermented foods as well, like natto and sauerkraut, and make sure you consume 20 percent of your calories from vegan-friendly protein, like seitan, tempeh, miso, and nuts and seeds. If you're vegetarian I recommend including pastured eggs and organic fermented dairy, including raw cheese, kefir, and yogurt. If you're pescatarian, include lots of wild-caught fish.

If you're a practicing vegan and struggling with low energy, doing a vegan-friendly version of my keto diet can give you what you need to restore your body to full health—without compromising your beliefs or your commitment to the planet. Here's what a sample day might look like:

7:30 a.m. Do a "spiritual triathlon": five minutes of gratitude practice, five minutes of reading the Bible or a book about personal growth, five minutes of prayer or meditation.

8:00 a.m. Drink a keto collagen smoothie with almond milk, 1 tablespoon of coconut oil, a scoop of bone broth protein or a scoop of vegan protein (on this plan I suggest using a small amount of animal-based protein for those who are open to it), ½ cup of berries, 1 teaspoon of cinnamon, and a scoop of antioxidant berry powder. Take your vitamin B supplement and probiotic.

9:00 a.m. Drink a cup of matcha green tea with a tablespoon of MCT oil.

12:00 p.m. Eat a large salad with vegetables, avocado, olive oil, and apple cider vinegar.

5:00 p.m. Exercise for at least 30 minutes. If you're just getting started with exercise, stick with walking for the first week or two. If you're accustomed to exercising, do your favorite activity—weight training, high-intensity interval training, running, biking, or yoga—for up to 60 minutes.

6:30 p.m. Eat a keto-friendly dinner. Take your probiotic.

8:00 p.m. Drink a glass of almond milk with a scoop of chocolate collagen protein and/or chocolate bone broth protein.

9:00 p.m. Turn off technology! Do something relaxing to prepare your brain for sleep: Read a book, write in your gratitude journal, take a warm bath with jasmine oil, meditate, or pray.

10:30 p.m. Lights out.

THE TOP FOUR SUPPLEMENTS TO SUPPORT THE KETO VEGAN PLAN

1. **B_{12} or B complex**. B_{12} deficiency is common in vegans. Diets that are dangerously low in this important vitamin can cause anemia because B_{12} helps produce healthy levels of red blood cells. B_{12} deficiency can also put you at risk of nervous system damage because the vitamin helps maintain the health of nerve cells. But even moderately low consumption of B_{12} can affect your mood, energy level, memory, skin, and digestion as well as increase your risk of heart disease and contribute to complications during pregnancy. B_{12} isn't found in most vegan foods, except in sources that are fortified, like some breakfast cereals, plant milks, and soy products. Studies have shown that the B_{12} in blue-green algae is among the least absorbable sources, so it's not safe to rely on algae alone. Since you can't eat fortified cereals on the keto

diet, it's smart to take a supplement. No one needs large quantities of B_{12}, but we do need to replenish our supply every day. B vitamins are water soluble and flushed out of the body easily. Adults should get 2.4 micrograms a day. Pregnant women should get 2.6 micrograms and women who are breastfeeding should get 2.8.

2. **Keto collagen, multicollagen protein, or vegan protein.** I advised Claire to take a collagen supplement because she was suffering from knee pain, and adequate collagen is needed for strong bones, joints, and skin. I believe it's a good option even if you're not having joint pain, because maintaining collagen levels is essential to prevent age-related decline—and levels decrease as we get older. In order to take this supplement, however, you need to be willing to consume a small quantity of animal-based collagen. If that doesn't sound appealing, I highly advise that you consume a vegan protein supplement. On the keto diet, you can't have beans, lentils, or peas, which makes it difficult for vegans to meet their protein needs—and protein is vital for maintaining muscle mass. Add a scoop of vegan protein powder to your morning smoothie to ensure you're getting adequate protein.

3. **Probiotics.** These nutritious supplements not only are great for your gut, but also help you produce and digest B vitamins. The health of your digestive system is an important factor in your ability to absorb adequate levels of B_{12}. Many people absorb only about 50 percent of the vitamin B_{12} they consume from food sources, and sometimes much less. Taking probiotics is advisable for many reasons—but when you're eating a vegan diet, it's especially vital to support your absorption of B_{12}. Take 50 billion CFU one or two times a day.

4. **Vitamin C or camu camu.** The best way to support your body's own collagen production is to consume real collagen from bone broth or in supplement form. But making sure you get enough vitamin C–rich foods in your diet can also support collagen growth. Taking 1 tablespoon daily of a powdered form of organic, low-sugar, vitamin C–rich superfruits like camu camu or amla berry is beneficial as well.

Other ancient remedies that may support vegans on my keto diet program include adaptogenic herbs like schisandra, fo-ti, rehmannia, ashwagandha, and the medicinal mushroom reishi.

SAMPLE SEVEN-DAY MEAL PLAN

Day 1

Breakfast

   Keto Pancakes★ (page 236)

   Herbal tea

Lunch

   Chicken Salad Lettuce Wraps★ (page 245)

   ½ avocado

Snack (optional)

   Celery sticks served with 1 tablespoon of *Cinnamon Nut Butter*
   (page 276)

Dinner

   Zucchini noodles topped with cherry tomatoes and avocado sauce
   (avocado, lemon juice, pine nuts, water, and seasonings to taste)

   ½ cup of mixed berries

Day 2

Breakfast

   Blueberry Smoothie (page 240)

Lunch

   Raw walnut tacos (made with raw walnuts, coconut aminos,
   seasonings to taste, and romaine lettuce leaves) served with
   guacamole

   ½ cup of strawberries

Snack (optional)

   Keto Fat Bomb (page 279)

Dinner

   Spaghetti and Marinara Meat Sauce★ (page 253)

★Note: See this recipe's "Make It Vegan" option.

Kale salad (2 cups of kale, 1 tablespoon of olive oil, ½ tablespoon of lemon juice, 2 tablespoons of pine nuts, and 1 tablespoon of dried cranberries)

Dessert

Keto Brownie★ (page 290)

Day 3

Breakfast

1 cup of *Granola* (page 283) served with ½ cup of almond milk and ½ cup of blueberries
Herbal tea

Lunch

Leftover *Spaghetti and Marinara Meat Sauce*★ (page 253)

Snack (optional)

6 ounces of raspberries served with 1 tablespoon of almond butter

Dinner

Chicken Vegetable Soup★ (page 250)
Side salad

Day 4

Breakfast

Yogurt parfait (made with leftover *Granola* [page 283], unsweetened coconut yogurt, fresh berries, unsweetened shredded coconut, almond butter, and cacao nibs)
Herbal tea

Lunch

Strawberry Spinach Salad with Poppy Seed Dressing★ (page 270)

Snack (optional)

½ avocado

★Note: See this recipe's "Make It Vegan" option.

Dinner

 Vegetarian Ceviche with Mushrooms (page 259)

 5 ounces of steamed kale topped with 1 to 2 tablespoons of olive oil
 and seasoned to taste

Dessert

 Peppermint Patty (page 285)

Day 5

Breakfast

 Turmeric Smoothie (page 241)

Lunch

 Leftover *Vegetarian Ceviche with Mushrooms* (page 259)

 ½ avocado

Snack (optional)

 Kale Chips (page 281)

Dinner

 Cauliflower Steak (page 261)

 6 ounces of green beans sautéed in 1 to 2 tablespoons of coconut oil
 and seasoned to taste

 ¼ cup of blueberries

Day 6

Breakfast

 Chia Pudding (page 279)

 Herbal tea

Lunch

 Avocado stuffed with diced tomatoes, cucumbers, bell peppers,
 onion, and *Tahini Lemon Dressing* (page 275)

 Side salad

 ½ cup of raspberries

*Note: See this recipe's "Make It Vegan" option.

Snack (optional)

½ avocado

Dinner

Zucchini Lasagna★ (page 264)

Side salad

Dessert

Toasted Coconut Macaroon (page 289)

Day 7

Breakfast

Scrambled tofu (tofu, spinach, mushrooms, cherry tomatoes, and
seasonings to taste and cooked in coconut oil)

Herbal tea

Lunch

Leftover Zucchini Lasagna★ (page 264)

Snack (optional)

½ cup of strawberries served with 1 tablespoon of almond butter

Dinner

Mashed Caul-tatoes (page 269)

Cucumber Salad with Tomato and Onion (page 270)

9 ounces of grilled asparagus drizzled with 1 to 2 tablespoons of
olive oil and seasoned to taste

★Note: See this recipe's "Make It Vegan" option.

CHAPTER 14

The Keto Collagen-Boosting Plan

Maximizing the Diet's Age-Defying and Beauty-Enhancing Benefits

From the time she was a kid, my sister, Rachel, has been disappointed by the fact that she couldn't grow her nails and her hair didn't have the thickness or luster of many of her friends'. She figured she'd be stuck with those problems forever—and feared that they would only get worse with age. But two years ago, she called me, sounding excited. She told me she'd started having 2 to 3 scoops of collagen and bone broth protein every day, both of which build healthy collagen and work well together if you're looking to maximize your collagen intake, and was eating more vitamin C–rich foods like citrus, goji berries, broccoli, and bell peppers. After just a month, she was able to grow her fingernails for the first time in her life. What's more, when she went to her longtime hair stylist, the woman commented on how much thicker her hair was. Even her skin looked better.

Rachel was deficient in collagen—and she's not alone. Collagen is the most abundant structural protein in our bodies. It's found in muscles, bones, skin, hair, nails, ligaments, tendons, blood vessels, organs, and the digestive tract. It gives our skin strength and elasticity. It's the main component of connective tissue, like ligaments and tendons. It's the glue that holds the body together.

We manufacture collagen from amino acids in protein-rich foods.

Other nutrients, like vitamins C and A, play an important role in the process as well. But as we age, collagen production naturally begins to slow, resulting in wrinkles, sagging skin, brittle nails, thinning hair, and joint pain. Eating a diet high in sugar, smoking, and getting too much sun can exacerbate the problem. Fortunately, studies show that adding collagen to your diet can help turn some of the age-related problems around.

For instance, a number of studies have shown that collagen supplements can have an antiaging effect on skin. In one double-blind, placebo-controlled trial published in *Skin Pharmacology and Physiology*, a group of women taking a collagen supplement once a day for eight weeks were compared to women who were given a placebo.[1] At the end of the study, the women in the collagen group had significant improvement in the elasticity of their skin. Another study found that after eight weeks a collagen supplement led to a noticeable reduction in skin dryness, wrinkles, and the depth of the nasolabial fold—the smile lines that run between your nose and mouth and usually deepen with age—and after twelve weeks it led to an increase in skin firmness.[2] A 2017 study helped explain why. It found that collagen is transferred through the bloodstream directly to the skin.[3]

Collagen may also help people with brittle nails, according to a study published in the *Journal of Cosmetic Dermatology*.[4] Other research in the *Journal of Investigative Dermatology* hints at the fact that it might help with hair-follicle regeneration.[5]

Studies have also revealed that collagen can be helpful for knee pain. One study of men and women over fifty who suffer from joint pain found that more than half of those who took collagen supplements for six months had a statistically significant improvement of 20 percent or more.[6] Another twenty-four-week study published in *Current Medical Research and Opinion* looked at 147 young athletes with joint pain.[7] Some received a daily collagen supplement and the rest received a placebo. By the end of the study, the participants who had taken the collagen had less joint pain at rest, when walking, when standing, when carrying objects, and when lifting. And researchers at Beth Israel Hospital in Boston found that supplementing with type 2 collagen, which is found in cartilage, helped patients suffering from rheumatoid arthritis find relief from painful symptoms by decreasing swelling in tender joints.[8]

Meanwhile, there's evidence that taking a gelatin supplement (which contains the same proteins as collagen), along with vitamin C (which helps your body synthesize collagen) before brief, intensive exercise can help build ligaments, tendons, and bones. Collagen can also improve your all-important gut health by "sealing and healing" the protective lining of your digestive tract.

Most of these studies looked at people taking one serving of collagen a day. I've seen remarkable benefits from a thirty-day collagen-loading program that includes three servings a day. (Another quick-start option is my 3-Day Keto Collagen Cleanse Plan. Find it at www.draxe.com/keto-diet-collagen.)

Here are the five easiest ways to get those servings in:

1 cup of homemade or frozen bone broth

1 scoop of a multicollagen supplement that contains types 1, 2, 3, 5, and 10

1 scoop of keto-optimized collagen

1 scoop of bone broth protein

Two servings of salmon or chicken skin (a serving is the equivalent of the skin on the leg, thigh, and breast)

To help you get started on the keto collagen plan, here's what a sample day might look like:

7:30 a.m. Do a "spiritual triathlon": five minutes of gratitude practice, five minutes of reading the Bible or a book about personal growth, five minutes of prayer or meditation.

8:00 a.m. Drink a keto collagen smoothie with almond milk, 1 tablespoon of coconut oil, a scoop of bone broth protein, a scoop of multicollagen protein, ½ cup of berries, 1 teaspoon of cinnamon, and a scoop of antioxidant berry powder.

9:00 a.m. Drink a cup of matcha green tea or black coffee with 1 tablespoon of MCT oil.

12:00 p.m. Eat a large salad with organic chicken, vegetables, olive oil, avocado, and apple cider vinegar.

5:00 p.m. Exercise for at least 30 minutes. If you're just getting started with exercise, stick with walking for the first week or two. If you're accustomed to exercising, do your favorite activity—weight training, high-intensity interval training, running, biking, or yoga—for up to 60 minutes.

6:30 p.m. Eat a keto-friendly dinner.

8:00 p.m. Drink a glass of almond milk with a scoop of collagen protein and bone broth protein. The flavored options, chocolate or vanilla, make this extra tasty.

9:00 p.m. Turn off technology! Do something relaxing to prepare your brain for sleep: Read a book, write in your gratitude journal, take a warm bath with jasmine oil, meditate, or pray.

10:30 p.m. Lights out.

THE TOP THREE SUPPLEMENTS TO SUPPORT YOUR KETO COLLAGEN-BOOSTING PLAN

1. **Keto-optimized collagen** contains the precise combination of macronutrients you need to stay in ketosis, plus a healthy serving of collagen. Look for a product that contains a combination of collagen along with healthy fats like MCT oil. If you can't have keto-optimized collagen, look for a multicollagen protein mixed with coconut or MCT oil. Add a scoop to your smoothie, green drink, or coffee once or twice a day.

2. **Bone broth protein** is another helpful supplement because of its high levels of type 1, 2, and 3 collagen. Also, protein powders made from bone broth are extremely high in collagen-boosting compounds, including hyaluronic acid, glucosamine, and chondroitin, so you reap additional benefits. Add a scoop to your favorite keto beverage once or twice a day.

3. **Superberry powder**, like camu camu or amla berry, will promote your body's natural collagen production because it's high in vitamin C. Look for berry powders that are certified organic. Because

fruits rich in vitamin C are sour, they make a good base for healthy lemonade. Just mix a scoop into a glass of water with a pinch of stevia.

Sample Seven-Day Meal Plan

Day 1

Breakfast
> *Keto Collagen Shake* (page 240)
> *Keto Coffee* (page 244) or tea/herbal infusion of your choice

Lunch
> *Chicken Salad Lettuce Wraps* (page 245)
> Sliced bell peppers and hummus
> Herbal infusion/tea

Snack (optional)
> Guacamole served with fresh veggies

Dinner
> 6 ounces of wild-caught salmon (or another type of wild-caught fish) cooked in 1 tablespoon of coconut or olive oil
> Steamed broccoli or Brussels sprouts topped with 1 tablespoon of flax oil and seasoned to taste
> ¼ cup of blackberries
> Herbal infusion/tea

Day 2

Breakfast
> *Low Carb Egg Muffin* (page 237)
> *Keto Coffee* (page 244) or tea/herbal infusion of your choice

Lunch
> Chicken vegetable bone broth soup (chicken broth, chicken, carrots, celery, onions, parsley, and sea salt)
> Side salad
> Herbal infusion/tea

Snack (optional)

½ cup of strawberries served with 1 tablespoon of almond butter

Dinner

6 ounces of organic, grass-fed bison cooked in 2 tablespoons of
coconut oil

Mashed Caul-tatoes (page 269)

Sautéed Spinach (page 267)

Herbal infusion/tea

Dessert

Keto Brownie (page 290)

Day 3

Breakfast

Blueberry Smoothie (page 240)

Keto Coffee (page 244) or tea/herbal infusion of your choice

Lunch

Strawberry Spinach Salad with Poppy Seed Dressing (page 270)

Herbal infusion/tea

Snack (optional)

Fresh veggies served with *Cinnamon Nut Butter* (page 276)

Dinner

Turkey Meatball Soup (page 251)

Side salad

Herbal infusion/tea

Day 4

Breakfast

Grain-Free Quiche (page 238)

Keto Coffee (page 244) or tea/herbal infusion of your choice

Lunch

Leftover *Turkey Meatball Soup* (page 251)

½ cup of fermented veggies

Herbal infusion/tea

Snack

1 ounce of goat cheese with celery sticks

Dinner

Salmon Cakes with Garlic Aioli (page 255)

9 ounces of asparagus drizzled with 1 to 2 tablespoons of olive oil
and seasoned to taste

Herbal infusion/tea

Dessert

Keto Chocolate Frosty (page 292)

Day 5

Breakfast

Keto Cashew Cookie Shake (page 242)

Keto Coffee (page 244) or tea/herbal infusion of your choice

Lunch

Leftover *Salmon Cakes with Garlic Aioli* (page 255)

Side salad

Herbal infusion/tea

Snack (optional)

Collagen-Boosting Blueberry Muffin (page 282)

Dinner

6 ounces of organic, free-range chicken cooked in 2 tablespoons of
coconut oil

6 ounces of summer squash sautéed in 1 to 2 tablespoons of ghee

Herbal infusion/tea

Day 6

Breakfast
> *Keto Pancakes* (page 236)
> *Keto Coffee* (page 244) or tea/herbal infusion of your choice

Lunch
> 6 ounces of organic, grass-fed lamb cooked in 2 tablespoons of
>   coconut oil
> 5 ounces of steamed kale topped with 1 to 2 tablespoons of olive oil
>   and seasoned to taste
> Herbal infusion/tea

Snack (optional)
> 1 ounce of goat cheese with celery sticks

Dinner
> *Thai Coconut Chicken Soup* (page 260)
> Side salad
> Herbal infusion/tea

Dessert
> *Toasted Coconut Macaroon* (page 289)

Day 7

Breakfast
> *Turmeric Smoothie* (page 241)
> *Keto Coffee* (page 244) or tea/herbal infusion of your choice

Lunch
> Leftover *Thai Coconut Chicken Soup* (page 260)
> Kale salad (2 cups of kale, 1 tablespoon of olive oil, ½ tablespoon of
>   lemon juice, 2 tablespoons of pine nuts, and 1 tablespoon of
>   dried cranberries)
> Herbal infusion/tea

Snack (optional)
> *Granola* (page 283) served with ½ cup of mixed berries

Dinner

6 ounces of organic, free-range chicken cooked in 1 tablespoon of
olive or coconut oil

Butter-Baked Brussels Sprouts (page 269)

Herbal infusion/tea

CHAPTER 15

The Keto Cancer Plan

Maximizing Your Diet's Disease-Fighting Power

Learning that you or a loved one has cancer is a frightening moment in anyone's life. But after going through that experience twice with my mom, as well as watching dear friends and loved ones weather the storm, I know there are a number of strategies that can help you stay strong in the face of this disease, both physically and mentally. Diet is one strategy that can help you get past cancer—and there's no diet that shows more promise than keto, especially when you do it the right way, with lots of nutrient-dense vegetables, herbs, and spices.

In Chapter 10, I provided a comprehensive overview of the medical literature showing the many ways in which the keto diet can be therapeutic for cancer. If you haven't read that yet and you or a loved one is considering using the keto approach for cancer, I suggest you flip to Chapter 10 and do so now. I won't reiterate that research here except to emphasize the bottom line: Because many types of tumors can use only glucose for fuel, by shifting your body from sugar burning to fat burning with ketosis, you slash cancer's source of sustenance, giving you a better shot at shrinking tumors and beating the disease entirely.

But when it comes to cancer, "diet" includes your mind, body, and spirit—not just the fare you feed your body but the ways in which you nourish your emotional well-being and your soul. I believe that your thoughts and your outlook can make a difference when it comes to battling scary diseases like cancer—and I'm not alone. According to the

Centers for Disease Control and Prevention, 69 percent of cancer patients say they pray for their health.[1] And a study in the American Cancer Society's peer-reviewed journal *Cancer* found that cancer patients who experienced a sense of meaning, peace, or transcendence through religious or spiritual beliefs reported feeling the fewest physical problems.[2] (The researchers defined "religion" as belonging to a religious organization and attending organized services and "spirituality" as having a connection to a force larger than oneself.)

That's a hopeful finding. If patients' beliefs make them feel better about their own health, they may be more likely to take better care of themselves, reach out to others for help, and do everything they can to fight the disease—all of which can help the body mobilize a robust immune response.

MY MOM'S ANTICANCER PLAN

When I talk about my mom's second bout with cancer, people often ask me exactly what she did to beat it. So one day I jotted down an outline of her typical day, along with the natural cancer treatments and strategies that she used to transform her health. It has now been fifteen years since she received her diagnosis, and my mom, at sixty-five, is completely healthy and in the best shape of her life. I believe that her diet, along with all the supportive strategies she embraced, helped her get well. Here's the outline of her typical day, which I urge you to follow as well. (For more details on how my mom beat cancer, see www .draxe.com/keto-diet-cancer-plan. At the end of this chapter you'll find a seven-day meal plan as well—plus tons more easy recipes in Chapter 17.)

> 8:00 a.m. Drink a glass of herbal tea (usually milk thistle, which is good for cleansing) with fresh squeezed lemon juice and take two probiotic capsules that contain soil-based organisms.
>
> 8:30 a.m. Do a "spiritual triathlon": ten minutes of gratitude, ten minutes of Bible or devotional reading, ten minutes of prayer or meditation

9:00 a.m. Consume a green drink with celery, cucumber, spinach, romaine, cabbage, avocado, and lemon, plus herbs and spices, such as ginger, parsley, cilantro, and turmeric. Herbs are the most potent form of edible medicine. Each delicate sprig is packed with powerful phytonutrients that can bolster your body's ability to fight cancer.

10:00 a.m. Exercise! Go for a walk in nature, take a yoga class, swim, ride a bike, or go to the gym and lift weights. When you have cancer, the emphasis should be on sheer enjoyment rather than intensity, so find activities that you love and that make you feel healthy, vibrant, and alive.

12:00 p.m. Eat a large superfood salad with salmon, spinach, romaine, avocado, olives, cucumber, tomato, extra virgin olive oil, and apple cider vinegar.

3:00 p.m. Drink another veggie juice.

5:00 p.m. Get a lymphatic massage. A number of studies have found that massage can reduce pain, anxiety, fatigue, nausea, and depression in cancer patients, and a pilot study published in *Psycho-Oncology* found that a twenty-minute massage was enough to promote a significant reduction in the stress hormone cortisol in cancer patients undergoing chemotherapy.[3] Or use this time for other alternative therapies, like an acupuncture or chiropractic session, or sitting in a hyperbaric oxygen chamber—all of which may bolster your body's defenses and help subdue the disease.

6:00 p.m. Eat a bowl of chicken vegetable bone broth soup, along with probiotic supplements, before a keto-friendly dinner. For dinner, have a 4-ounce portion of grass-fed bison or turkey along with loads of vegetables like cauliflower, broccoli, and carrots drizzled in coconut oil and baked in the oven.

After dinner. Watch a funny movie or TV show. We all know that laughter is a great way to relieve stress—and studies prove it. Research published in *Alternative Therapies in Health and Medicine* found that, compared to women who watched a tourism video, those who viewed a humorous video had lower stress levels—and their immune function increased, as measured by changes in the activity of natural killer cells, white blood cells that kill tumor cells.[4]

10:00 p.m. Take a warm bath with Epsom salts and lavender oil while listening to an audiotape of healing scriptures or a guided meditation.

THE TOP FIVE SUPPLEMENTS TO SUPPORT YOUR KETO CANCER PLAN

1. **Turmeric and other cancer-fighting and immune-boosting herbs**, like ginger, garlic, thyme, cayenne pepper, oregano, and parsley, can keep your body's defenses strong. Use them liberally on your food, or if you're taking them in capsule form, take 250 to 500 milligrams once or twice a day.

2. **Probiotics** can balance the bacteria in your gut and bolster your overall wellness. They have also been shown to be helpful in cancer patients who experience bowel problems as a result of treatment. Take 50 billion CFU one or two times a day.

3. **Organic powdered greens** for alkalizing support your immune system and detoxify your body. Look for a product that contains ingredients like spirulina, chlorella, juiced grasses, vegetables, superfruits, and herbs. Add 1 or 2 scoops daily to your favorite keto-friendly beverage.

4. **Medicinal mushrooms**, such as reishi, cordyceps, turkey tail, maitake, and lion's mane, have immune-boosting properties. These mushrooms have been used for millennia in traditional Chinese medicine to help heal a number of diseases. More recently, they've been found to activate the immune system's T cells, whose job it is to seek out and destroy abnormal cells. You can add organic mushrooms to your favorite keto recipes or take a supplement. Follow dosage instructions on the bottle.

5. **Frankincense and myrrh essential oils** contain potent anti-cancer compounds. Just rub 2 to 5 drops on the front and back of your

neck (they don't require a carrier oil), so you can also get the aroma-therapy benefits. For advanced treatment, dilute 1 drop of each oil in 4 ounces of water, along with 20 drops of turmeric essential oil, and take orally.

Other supplements with cancer-fighting benefits include vitamin D, vitamin C, zinc, astragalus, milk thistle, proteolytic enzymes, and green tea extract.

SAMPLE SEVEN-DAY MEAL PLAN

Day 1

Early Morning
Herbal tea

Midmorning
Veggie juice

Lunch
Strawberry Spinach Salad with Poppy Seed Dressing (page 270)

Snack
Veggie juice
Beef vegetable bone broth soup

Dinner
4 ounces of wild-caught halibut cooked in 2 tablespoons of coconut oil
6 ounces of steamed Brussels sprouts topped with 1 tablespoon of flax oil and seasoned to taste

Day 2

Early Morning
Herbal tea

Midmorning
Veggie juice

Lunch

Superfood salad made with salmon, spinach, romaine, avocado,
olives, cucumber, tomato, extra virgin olive oil, and apple cider
vinegar

½ avocado

Snack

Veggie juice

Thai Chicken Coconut Soup (page 260)

Dinner

4 ounces of organic, free-range chicken cooked in 2 tablespoons of
coconut oil

Steamed broccoli and cauliflower drizzled with 2 tablespoons of
tahini and sea salt

Day 3

Early Morning

Herbal tea

Midmorning

Veggie juice

Lunch

Egg Tahini Salad (page 248)

½ cup of blueberries

Snack

Veggie juice

Leftover beef vegetable bone broth soup

Dinner

Cauliflower Steak (page 261)

Cajun Collard Greens (page 273)

Celery sticks served with *Cinnamon Nut Butter* (page 276)

Day 4

Early Morning
　　Herbal tea

Midmorning
　　Veggie juice

Lunch
　　Zucchini noodles topped with cherry tomatoes and avocado sauce
　　　　(avocado, lemon juice, pine nuts, water, and seasonings to taste)
　　Side salad

Snack
　　Veggie juice
　　Leftover *Thai Chicken Coconut Soup* (page 260)

Dinner
　　Burrito bowl (cauliflower rice, black beans, bell peppers, avocado,
　　　　red onion, and chicken or beef, topped with olive oil and lime
　　　　juice)
　　Side salad

Day 5

Early Morning
　　Herbal tea

Midmorning
　　Veggie juice

Lunch
　　Salmon Salad (page 249)
　　½ cup of strawberries

Snack
　　Veggie juice
　　Chicken Vegetable Soup (page 250)

Dinner

> Chicken Pesto (page 256)
> Butter-Baked Brussels Sprouts (page 269)
> Cucumber Salad with Tomato and Onion (page 270)

Day 6

Early Morning

> Herbal tea

Midmorning

> Veggie juice

Lunch

> 4 to 6 ounces of tuna salad (wild-caught canned tuna with 2 to 3
> tablespoons of avocado mayo) served over a bed of mixed
> greens
> ½ cup of blueberries

Snack

> Veggie juice
> Leftover *Chicken Vegetable Soup* (page 250)

Dinner

> 4 ounces of grass-fed, organic bison cooked in 2 tablespoons of
> coconut oil
> 6 ounces of steamed Brussels sprouts topped with 1 tablespoon of
> flax oil and seasoned to taste
> *Mashed Caul-tatoes* (page 269)

Day 7

Early Morning

> Herbal tea

Midmorning

> Veggie juice

Lunch

> Superfood salad made with beef or chicken, spinach, romaine, avocado, olives, cucumber, tomato, extra virgin olive oil, and apple cider vinegar

Snack

> Veggie juice
>
> Beef vegetable bone broth soup

Dinner

> 4 ounces of organic, free-range turkey cooked in 2 tablespoons of sesame oil
>
> 5 ounces of steamed spinach topped with 1 tablespoon of olive oil and seasoned to taste
>
> 9 ounces of grilled asparagus drizzled with 1 to 2 tablespoons of olive oil and seasoned to taste

CHAPTER 16

The Forever Keto Cycling Plan

The Easy, Sustainable Way to Make the Keto Diet a Way of Life

Now that you've spent a full thirty or sixty days on my keto diet program, your body has completely adapted to burning fat for fuel. You've presumably lost weight and seen substantial improvements in your overall health. I'm thrilled that you've come this far. Now it's time to downshift and put your body into a comfortable gear that you can maintain for a lifetime.

The automobile metaphor fits perfectly for the Forever Keto Cycling Plan. The human body is meant to function like a hybrid car, alternating between burning fat and burning carbs for fuel. Our ancestors cycled naturally in and out of ketosis, depending on the quantity and type of food that was available. When you're utilizing fat, it's like tapping the car's battery for power—the cleanest, healthiest option. But avoiding carbs for the rest of your life isn't realistic for most people. By adopting the Forever Keto Cycling Plan, a hybrid approach that allows you to consciously fluctuate between carb burning and fat burning, it's easier to go the distance and maintain the benefits of ketosis for the long term.

The Forever Keto Cycling Plan is easy, healthy, and supremely flexible, so you can play with it and find the pattern of carb and keto days that works for you. The approach I recommend to patients (and the one that has worked for my wife, Chelsea) is a rotating three-day pattern: two keto days when you eat fewer than 30 grams of carbs, followed by one carb day with between 80 and 100 grams of carbs, or 30 grams three times a day. The standard dietary guidelines recommend 225 to 325 grams of carbs a day, so even on your carb days you're still well below that level. Try to avoid foods with added sugar or supersweet desserts, so you don't reawaken the sugar-craving beast. Stick with delicious low-sugar options — a nice serving of quinoa (1 cup has about 40 grams of carbs), a medium sweet potato (45 grams), a slice or two of whole-grain bread (12 grams per slice), 1 cup of oatmeal (27 grams), or a few pieces of fruit (a plum has 8 grams; a peach has 12). A sweet dessert now and again won't kill you. But strive to stay away from processed foods and added sugar as much as possible to avoid weight gain and maintain the health improvements you've achieved with keto.

On your carb days you'll be utilizing glucose for fuel, so you won't be in ketosis. But because your thirty days on my keto diet program primed your body to be able to use fat for energy, you'll shift easily back into ketosis by the second keto day. Hundreds of former patients, family, and friends find that keto cycling is an easy-to-manage, fully sustainable way to maintain their health, their weight, and their social lives — and I believe you will, too. As Chelsea says, "With most diets you have to spend a lot of time on food prep and planning. You have to adapt your lifestyle to fit the diet. But keto cycling is a diet you can adapt to fit your lifestyle."

DR. CHELSEA'S EXPERIENCE WITH KETO CYCLING

Before starting her keto journey, Chelsea was frustrated by her health. As a chiropractor, certified yoga instructor, strength and conditioning coach, and CrossFit athlete, she had always taken good care of her body. She ate a wholesome diet and exercised five or six days a week. But she was never able to get as lean as she wanted to be, and she wasn't willing to starve herself or adopt unhealthy strategies to achieve that goal. Then she tried keto and saw some results. But for her, the biggest results came

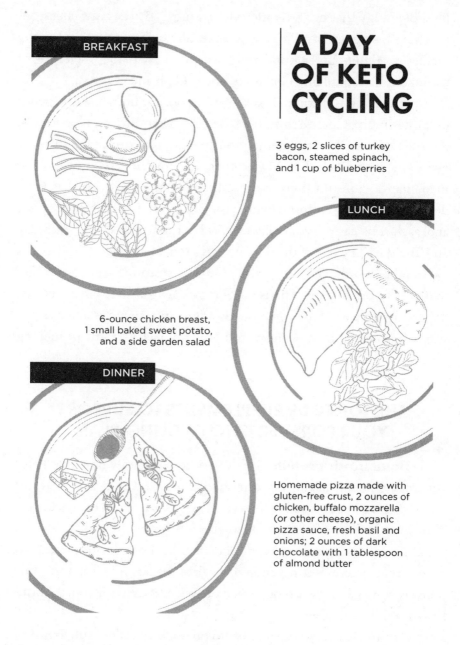

A DAY OF KETO CYCLING

BREAKFAST

3 eggs, 2 slices of turkey bacon, steamed spinach, and 1 cup of blueberries

LUNCH

6-ounce chicken breast, 1 small baked sweet potato, and a side garden salad

DINNER

Homemade pizza made with gluten-free crust, 2 ounces of chicken, buffalo mozzarella (or other cheese), organic pizza sauce, fresh basil and onions; 2 ounces of dark chocolate with 1 tablespoon of almond butter

during the first three months she did keto cycling. She lost ten pounds in all and reached her ideal weight and shape.

Her health improved, too. For years she had struggled with painful periods, but the keto diet balanced her hormones so she no longer has problems. And keto cycling allowed her to maintain the extraordinary level of energy that her busy lifestyle requires. (By the way, check out Chelsea's Instagram page @drchelseaaxe. She is always posting healthy recipes, workouts, and natural beauty tips along with lots of pictures of us and our Cavalier King Charles spaniels, Flash and Oakley.)

Keto cycling is flexible. If we're going out for dinner with friends on Friday night, Chelsea shifts her schedule so her carb day is on Friday. And she exercises more intensely on her carb days to make sure her energy doesn't take a hit. My brother, Dr. Jordan Axe, a functional medicine doctor and thyroid specialist in Tampa, Florida, has been doing keto cycling for more than a year, and he takes a slightly different approach. His carb days are always Friday night and all day Saturday and Tuesday. The rest of the time he eats a strict keto diet.

In other words, you can—and should—customize the eating plan to make it work for you. This is a program that's meant to last a lifetime. Tweaking it is part of the equation. So adjust and amend as much as you want. But *commit* to it—and you'll give yourself the gift of lifelong health.

THE TOP FOUR SUPPLEMENTS TO SUPPORT YOUR FOREVER KETO CYCLING PLAN

1. **Bone broth protein** gives you a keto-friendly base that helps you maintain the health of your gut, joints, and skin and provides superfuel for a healthy, active lifestyle. Take 1 scoop once or twice a day with your favorite smoothie or keto-friendly beverage.

2. **Keto collagen** works in tandem with bone broth protein to ensure that you're getting enough healthy collagen to support your body as you age. Take 1 scoop once or twice a day with your favorite keto-friendly beverage.

3. **Probiotics** keep your gut health on track and allow you to maintain a wholesome population of intestinal microbes as you add small amounts of carbs back into your diet. Take 50 billion CFU one or two times a day.

4. **A good multivitamin** with D_3, C (from sources like camu camu), K, an assortment of Bs, including B_{12}, as well as chromium and

selenium will ensure that you're closing any nutritional gaps. Multivitamin formulations vary, so take the standard dosage recommended on the bottle.

For more on how to use keto cycling, visit www.draxe.com/keto-diet-cycling-plan.

SAMPLE SEVEN-DAY MEAL PLAN

Day 1 — Keto Day

Breakfast

> 3 eggs and 2 slices of turkey bacon
> Steamed spinach
> *Keto Coffee* (page 244)

Lunch

> *Turkey Meatball Soup* (page 251)
> Side salad

Snack (optional)

> Celery sticks served with 2 tablespoons of hummus

Dinner

> Burrito bowl (cauliflower rice, black beans, bell peppers, avocado, red onion, and chicken or beef, topped with olive oil and lime juice)

Day 2 — Keto Day

Breakfast

> *Keto Cashew Cookie Shake* (page 242)

Lunch

> *Albacore Tuna Salad* (page 247) served over a bed of mixed greens
> ½ avocado, sliced

Snack (optional)

> Keto shake (1 scoop of keto protein powder, 1 cup of water, a handful of strawberries, and ice cubes)

Dinner

  Cauliflower Steak (page 261)

  Sautéed Spinach (page 267)

Day 3—Carb Day

Breakfast

  ½ cup of oatmeal with ½ banana, 1 scoop of vanilla collagen
    protein, and 2 tablespoons of chopped walnuts

Lunch

  6-ounce chicken breast

  1 small baked sweet potato

  Side garden salad

Snack (optional)

  1 slice *Keto Bread* (page 280)

Dinner

  Grass-fed beef burger in a lettuce wrap with tomato, ketchup, and
    mustard

  Side of steamed spinach

Dessert

  Keto Cheesecake (page 291)

Day 4—Keto Day

Breakfast

  Keto smoothie (1 scoop of vanilla or chocolate keto protein
    powder, 1 cup of coconut milk, and 2 tablespoons of
    hempseeds)

Lunch

  Large salad consisting of 4 ounces of chicken or grass-fed steak, ½
    avocado, mixed greens, sliced cucumber, diced tomato, and 2
    tablespoons of *Avocado Ranch Dressing* (page 276)

Snack (optional)

¼ cup of salted sprouted almonds

Dinner

Zucchini Lasagna (page 264)

Side salad

Day 5 — Keto Day

Breakfast

Keto Chocolate Smoothie (page 242)

Lunch

Salmon Salad (page 249)

Snack (optional)

Collagen-Boosting Blueberry Muffin (page 282)

Dinner

Coconut Chicken Tenders (page 258)

Steamed broccoli and cauliflower drizzled with 2 tablespoons of
tahini and sea salt

Day 6 — Carb Day

Breakfast

Keto Pancakes (page 236)

Turkey Breakfast Sausage (page 237)

Lunch

BLT Turkey Wrap (page 246) served on sprouted whole-grain bread

Side salad

Snack (optional)

1 ounce of goat cheese with celery sticks

Dinner

  Homemade pizza made with gluten-free crust, 2 ounces of
    chicken, buffalo mozzarella (or other cheese), organic pizza
    sauce, fresh basil, and onions

Dessert

  2 ounces of dark chocolate served with 1 tablespoon of almond
    butter

Day 7 — Keto Day

Breakfast

  Veggie Omelet (page 239)
  Turkey bacon
  Matcha green tea

Lunch

  Chicken salad in lettuce wraps
  Salad (romaine lettuce, turkey bacon bits, and tomato served with
    Cashew Caesar Dressing [page 275])

Snack (optional)

  ½ cup of goat's milk cottage cheese with a handful of berries

Dinner

  Lamb Burger (page 261)
  Steamed veggies
  ½ an avocado

BEST OF LUCK ON YOUR KETO JOURNEY

I couldn't be happier that you've chosen to embrace my keto diet program. By adopting this new approach to eating, you'll be able to achieve the health and weight goals you've always dreamed of—and, as your body heals, you'll experience an abundance of other good things: more energy, less pain, increased mental clarity, deeper happiness, a renewed ability to participate in the activities you've always enjoyed, and an enlarged capacity to share meaningful, active, joyful moments with friends and loved ones. These are the things that lie ahead as you make keto a way of life—and the things I wish for you as you move through this program in the months and years ahead. I'm grateful to you for choosing this path. May you find healing, health, and peace.

Blessings,

Dr. Axe

PART IV

Keto Diet Eating

CHAPTER 17

Keto Diet Recipes

This chapter features more than eighty of my most delicious keto-friendly recipes. You'll find everything from my favorite energy-boosting smoothies to grab-and-go breakfast options to dinner recipes such as steak and lasagna. And you won't believe how great the decadent Keto Pancakes are! You won't miss those carb-laden options.

When you're shopping for ingredients, keep in mind that for the greatest health benefits, you should always choose organic. Remember to opt for grass-fed beef, pasture-raised poultry, and wild-caught fish as well. Your local supermarket should have some great staples in the organic section and even in the conventional baking section, but you may need to visit your local health food or supplement stores (or shop online) for a few select ingredients such as the collagen and protein powders.

BREAKFASTS, SMOOTHIES, AND DRINKS

KETO PANCAKES

SERVINGS: 4 TO 5 (2 PANCAKES PER SERVING)
TIME: 20 MINUTES

¾ cup almond flour

¼ cup coconut flour

1 scoop vanilla bone broth protein or keto collagen powder

1 teaspoon baking powder

¼ teaspoon sea salt

3 eggs

¼ cup coconut cream

1 teaspoon monk-fruit sweetener

3 tablespoons water

1 tablespoon coconut oil, melted

¼ cup almond butter (optional)

In a large bowl, mix together the almond flour, coconut flour, bone broth protein, baking powder, and sea salt. Set aside.

In a medium bowl, beat together the eggs, coconut cream, and monk-fruit sweetener with a fork or whisk. Beat for 30 seconds for ultimate fluffiness.

Incorporate the egg mixture into the flour mixture, stirring well.

Add the water and coconut oil and stir until the batter thickens.

In a large greased skillet over medium heat, add the batter by the spoonful.

Let each pancake sit for 3 to 4 minutes before flipping. They are ready to flip when they are easily lifted from the pan with a spatula.

Flip and cook for another 2 to 3 minutes.

Melt the almond butter (if using) and pour over the top.

Make It Vegan

Replace the eggs with 3 tablespoons flaxseed powder and ½ cup water.

Omit the bone broth protein or keto collagen powder.

Add 2 more tablespoons water and 1 more tablespoon coconut oil.

TURKEY BREAKFAST SAUSAGE

SERVINGS: 3 TO 4 (2 PATTIES PER SERVING)

TIME: 15 MINUTES

2 teaspoons dried sage

2 teaspoons sea salt

1/2 teaspoon ground black pepper

1/2 teaspoon red pepper flakes

1/4 teaspoon garlic powder

1 pound ground turkey

1 tablespoon avocado oil

Using your hands, mix all of the spices into the ground turkey.

In a medium to large skillet over medium heat, add the avocado oil.

Form the meat into 6 to 8 round, flat patties and carefully place them in the hot skillet with a spatula.

Cook each patty for 3 to 4 minutes on each side, or until cooked through.

LOW-CARB EGG MUFFINS

SERVINGS: 6

TIME: 20 MINUTES

6 eggs

1/4 cup unsweetened almond milk

1/4 cup shredded Parmesan cheese

Sea salt and ground black pepper, to taste

Preheat the oven to 375°F.

In a medium bowl, beat together the eggs and almond milk.

Divide the egg mixture among 6 of the cups in a greased or lined muffin pan, filling the cups about three-quarters of the way.

Top with the Parmesan cheese, salt, and pepper.

Bake for 15 minutes and serve immediately.

Make It Dairy-Free

Omit the Parmesan or use a dairy-free cheese.

Give It a Collagen Boost

Add 1 scoop of collagen protein to the egg mixture.

GRAIN-FREE QUICHE

SERVINGS: 6 TO 8

TIME: 1 HOUR

CRUST:

1¾ cups almond meal

¼ cup coconut flour

1 garlic clove, minced

1 teaspoon dried oregano

Pinch of sea salt

⅓ cup avocado or olive oil

2 tablespoons water

FILLING:

1 tablespoon avocado or olive oil

2 garlic cloves, minced

1 cup cremini or button mushrooms, thinly sliced

½ shallot, sliced

6 large eggs

⅓ cup unsweetened almond milk

½ teaspoon sea salt

2 ounces goat cheese, crumbled

Preheat the oven to 400°F.

In a medium bowl, combine all the crust ingredients. Mix well until the dough becomes crumbly.

Place the dough in a greased 9-inch pie pan and with clean hands press it out over the bottom of the pan and 1 to 1¼ inches up the sides of the pan.

Bake for 15 minutes.

Meanwhile, in a medium skillet over medium heat, heat the avocado oil. Sauté the garlic, mushrooms, and shallot for 5 minutes. Set aside to cool.

In a large bowl, beat the eggs and almond milk. Add the sea salt and gently stir in the vegetable mixture and goat cheese.

Pour the filling into the baked crust, reduce the oven temperature to 375°F, and bake for another 30 minutes, or until the eggs are cooked through.

Slice and serve. Leftovers can be stored in the refrigerator for up to 2 days.

Make It Dairy-Free

Use an alternative plant-based goat "cheese," or omit the cheese altogether.

Give It a Collagen Boost

Add 1 scoop of collagen protein to the beaten eggs before adding the vegetable mixture.

VEGGIE OMELET

SERVINGS: 1
TIME: 10 MINUTES

1 garlic clove, minced
½ cup chopped red bell pepper
½ cup chopped green bell pepper
½ cup chopped mushrooms
¼ cup chopped red onion
2 tablespoons grass-fed butter
3 eggs
2 ounces raw cheese
Dried oregano, sliced fresh chives, sea salt, and black pepper, to taste

In a large skillet over medium-low heat, sauté the garlic, peppers, mushrooms, and onion in the butter for 5 minutes.

In a small bowl, beat the eggs and add to the skillet.

Shred the cheese on top and fold into an omelet.

Serve topped with the oregano, chives, sea salt, and black pepper.

BLUEBERRY SMOOTHIE

SERVINGS: I
TIME: 5 MINUTES

½ cup full-fat coconut milk

½ cup fresh baby spinach

½ cup frozen wild blueberries

I scoop keto collagen powder

I tablespoon almond butter

Place all the ingredients in a high-speed blender and blend until smooth.

Make It Vegan

Omit the keto collagen powder and add I tablespoon coconut oil.

KETO COLLAGEN SHAKE

SERVINGS: I
TIME: 5 MINUTES

I cup full-fat coconut milk

¼ cup cold water

I scoop collagen protein

I scoop vanilla bone broth protein

I tablespoon goji berry powder

Pour the coconut milk and water into a high-speed blender.

Add the collagen protein, vanilla bone broth protein, and goji berry powder.

Blend on low speed until smooth.

TURMERIC SMOOTHIE

SERVINGS: I
TIME: 5 MINUTES

¾ cup full-fat coconut milk
¼ cup unsweetened almond milk
1 teaspoon ground turmeric
½ teaspoon ground ginger
¼ teaspoon ground cinnamon
¼ teaspoon ground black pepper
1 scoop collagen protein
5 drops liquid stevia
5 to 6 ice cubes
½ frozen avocado

Place all the ingredients, except the ice cubes and avocado, in a high-speed blender. Pulse several times.

Add the ice cubes and avocado and blend on high until smooth.

Make It Vegan

Omit the collagen protein and add a plant-based keto protein powder.

VANILLA BEAN SMOOTHIE

SERVINGS: I
TIME: 5 MINUTES

1 cup full-fat coconut milk
½ teaspoon pure vanilla extract
1 scoop vanilla bone broth protein
½ cup water
1 cup ice
Pinch of sea salt
2 to 3 drops liquid stevia (optional)

Place all the ingredients in a high-speed blender and blend until smooth.

KETO CASHEW COOKIE SHAKE

SERVINGS: 1
TIME: 5 MINUTES

1 cup full-fat coconut or unsweetened almond milk

1 scoop chocolate keto protein powder (or collagen protein plus 1
tablespoon MCT oil) or chocolate bone broth protein

1 tablespoon cacao powder

2 tablespoons cashew butter (or peanut or almond butter)

1/8 teaspoon pumpkin pie spice

Place all the ingredients in a high-speed blender and blend until
smooth.

KETO CHOCOLATE SMOOTHIE

SERVINGS: 1 TO 2
TIME: 5 MINUTES

1/2 cup unsweetened almond milk

1 tablespoon coconut oil

1 tablespoon almond butter

1 scoop chocolate keto protein powder (or collagen protein plus 1
tablespoon MCT oil) or chocolate bone broth protein

4 to 6 ice cubes

Place all the ingredients in a high-speed blender and blend until
smooth.

KETO GREEN SMOOTHIE

SERVINGS: 1 TO 2
TIME: 5 MINUTES

1 cup unsweetened almond milk
1/2 cucumber
1/2 avocado
1 cup fresh spinach
1 teaspoon matcha
2 celery stalks
1 tablespoon chia seeds
1 scoop vanilla keto protein powder (or collagen protein plus 1
    tablespoon MCT oil)

Place all the ingredients in a high-speed blender and blend until smooth.

Make It Vegan

Replace the keto protein powder with 5 to 6 drops liquid stevia.

PROBIOTIC KEFIR SMOOTHIE

SERVINGS: 2
TIME: 5 MINUTES

1 cup kefir (coconut milk kefir or goat's milk kefir)
1 scoop vanilla bone broth protein or vanilla collagen protein
1/2 frozen avocado
1 tablespoon cashew or almond butter
1 tablespoon coconut oil
1/4 cup water
Ice (optional)
Ground cinnamon, to taste

Place all the ingredients except the cinnamon in a high-speed blender and blend until smooth.
Top with cinnamon.

KETO COFFEE

SERVINGS: 1
TIME: 5 MINUTES

1 (8-ounce) cup coffee
1 scoop vanilla keto protein powder or collagen protein
1 to 2 tablespoons grass-fed butter or ghee

Place all the ingredients in a high-speed blender and blend until well combined.

TURMERIC GOLDEN MILK

SERVINGS: 2
TIME: 10 MINUTES

3 cups unsweetened almond milk
2 tablespoons coconut cream
2 teaspoons ground turmeric
1 teaspoon ground ginger
1/2 teaspoon ground black pepper
2 cinnamon sticks (or 1 teaspoon ground cinnamon)
2 tablespoons coconut oil or ghee
5 to 6 drops liquid stevia

Place the almond milk, coconut cream, turmeric, ginger, and black pepper in a high-speed blender. Pulse several times.

Pour the milk mixture from the blender into a small saucepan and heat over medium heat until near boiling. Reduce the heat to low at the first sign of a boil.

Stir in the cinnamon sticks, coconut oil, and stevia. Stir, cover, and let simmer for 5 minutes.

Discard the cinnamon sticks, stir again, and serve immediately. Store any leftovers in the refrigerator for up to 2 days.

MAIN DISHES

CHICKEN SALAD LETTUCE WRAPS

SERVINGS: 4
TIME: 15 MINUTES

CHICKEN SALAD:

1 cooked rotisserie chicken
2 celery stalks, diced
½ cup avocado oil mayonnaise
¼ cup pecans, chopped
2 teaspoons apple cider vinegar
¼ teaspoon sea salt
¼ teaspoon ground black pepper

LETTUCE WRAP ASSEMBLY:

4 leaves butter lettuce
1 avocado, cubed
2 Roma tomatoes, diced

Pick and chop or shred the meat from the rotisserie chicken.

In a large bowl, add the chicken and the rest of the ingredients and mix well.

Fill each of the leaves with about ½ cup chicken salad. Top with the avocado and tomatoes.

Make It Vegan:
Use shredded jackfruit instead of chicken.

Give It a Collagen Boost:
Stir 1 scoop of collagen protein into the chicken salad.

KETO BEEF TACOS IN ROMAINE BOATS

SERVINGS: 4
TIME: 20 MINUTES

8 ounces grass-fed ground beef
1 (10-ounce) jar diced fire-roasted tomatoes, drained
1/2 white onion, sliced
2 tablespoons cream cheese
8 romaine lettuce leaves, doubled up for serving
Spinach or leafy greens of choice
4 green onions, sliced
1 avocado, sliced
Sprouts, to taste

In a medium pan over medium heat, add the ground beef and cook until nearly browned. Add the tomatoes and sliced onions. Use a wooden spatula or spoon to stir until well combined.

Once the onions are translucent, add the cream cheese and continue stirring until the cream cheese has melted into the beef mixture.

Place the beef mixture in the romaine lettuce leaves and top with spinach or leafy greens of choice, sliced green onions, sliced avocado, and sprouts.

BLT TURKEY WRAP

SERVINGS: 4
TIME: 10 MINUTES

1/2 cup avocado oil mayonnaise
1 teaspoon dried basil
1/2 teaspoon sea salt
1/4 teaspoon ground black pepper
8 romaine lettuce leaves
1 pound sliced turkey breast
8 slices turkey bacon, cooked
2 Roma tomatoes, sliced

In a small bowl, combine the mayonnaise, basil, sea salt, and pepper.

Spread equal portions of the mixture on the inside of each lettuce leaf.

Add equal portions of the turkey breast, bacon, and tomatoes to each.

Eat like a taco and enjoy.

ALBACORE TUNA SALAD

SERVINGS: 4

TIME: 5 MINUTES

2 (5-ounce) cans albacore tuna packed in water, drained

1/4 cup avocado oil mayonnaise

2 teaspoons Dijon mustard

2 teaspoons dried dill

2 teaspoons lime juice

1/2 cup diced bell pepper

Mixed greens

In a small bowl, combine the tuna, mayonnaise, mustard, dill, lime juice, and bell pepper.

Serve on a bed of mixed greens.

Give It a Collagen Boost

Add 1 scoop of collagen protein.

TURKEY SALAD

SERVINGS: 4
TIME: 10 MINUTES

1 pound turkey breast, cooked
3 green onions, sliced
2 celery stalks, diced
½ cup walnuts
½ cup avocado oil mayonnaise
1 teaspoon lemon juice
¼ teaspoon sea salt
¼ teaspoon ground black pepper
Mixed greens

Chop the turkey breast into small pieces.

In a large bowl, combine the turkey, onions, celery, walnuts, mayonnaise, lemon juice, salt, and pepper and mix well.

Serve on a bed of mixed greens.

Give It a Collagen Boost

Add 1 scoop of collagen protein.

EGG TAHINI SALAD

SERVINGS: 4
TIME: 5 MINUTES

4 cups fresh greens
2 Roma tomatoes, diced
1 bell pepper, diced
½ cup sliced radishes
1 avocado, sliced
6 hard-boiled eggs
2 ounces *Tahini Lemon Dressing* (page 275)

In a large bowl, place the greens, tomatoes, bell pepper, radishes, and avocado.

Slice, chop, or quarter the eggs and place them on top of the salad. Drizzle with the dressing and serve in individual bowls.

SALMON SALAD

SERVINGS: I
TIME: I5 MINUTES

I teaspoon coconut oil

4 ounces wild-caught salmon

¼ teaspoon sea salt

2 cups fresh greens

¼ cup sliced bell pepper

2 radishes, thinly sliced

¼ cup snap peas

½ avocado, diced

2 ounces *Tahini Lemon Dressing* (page 275), *Cashew Caesar Dressing* (page 275), or *Avocado Ranch Dressing* (page 276)

Turn the broiler on high.

In a medium oven-safe skillet over medium-high heat, add the coconut oil. Place the salmon skin side down in the skillet.

Cook the salmon for 4 to 5 minutes, flip, sprinkle with the sea salt, and move to the broiler. Cook for 6 minutes.

Meanwhile, in a large bowl, combine the greens, pepper, radishes, snap peas, and avocado.

Top the salad with the cooked salmon and drizzle with the desired dressing.

CHICKEN VEGETABLE SOUP

SERVINGS: 6 TO 8

TIME: 45 MINUTES

2 tablespoons avocado oil

2 garlic cloves, minced

½ large onion, diced

1 bell pepper, diced

2 celery stalks, diced

1 (32-ounce) carton free-range chicken bone broth

4 cups water

2 tablespoons apple cider vinegar

1 pound chicken breast

1 (15-ounce) can diced tomatoes with green chilies, undrained

2 cups green beans, fresh or frozen

1 teaspoon sea salt

2 bay leaves

1 small bunch fresh thyme

2 cups shredded kale

In a large soup pot over medium heat, add the avocado oil. Sauté the garlic, onion, bell pepper, and celery for 5 minutes.

Pour in the chicken broth, water, and apple cider vinegar. Stir well.

Add the remaining ingredients, except the kale.

Bring to a boil, reduce the heat to low, and cover. Allow to simmer for 25 minutes, or until the chicken has cooked through.

Carefully remove and shred the chicken breast using two forks, and then add it back to the soup.

Remove the bay leaves and thyme, and stir in the kale. Add more sea salt to taste. Once the kale has wilted a bit, the soup is ready to serve.

Make It Vegan

Omit the chicken and use vegetable broth in place of the chicken bone broth.

TURKEY MEATBALL SOUP

SERVINGS: 6 TO 8

TIME: 1 HOUR, 10 MINUTES

MEATBALLS:

1 pound ground turkey

1 tablespoon coconut flour

½ cup finely chopped fresh parsley

2 eggs

½ teaspoon sea salt

½ teaspoon garlic powder

SOUP:

¼ cup avocado oil

4 celery stalks, diced

1 sweet onion, diced

1 bell pepper, diced

2 garlic cloves, minced

1 (32-ounce) carton free-range chicken stock

2 cups water

1 (28-ounce) can diced tomatoes

1 tablespoon Italian seasoning

1 teaspoon sea salt

2 cups fresh shredded kale or spinach

¼ cup finely chopped fresh parsley

Preheat the oven to 400°F.

In a large bowl, combine all the meatball ingredients. Mix with clean hands.

Line a rimmed baking sheet with parchment paper. Using a tablespoon, scoop out the meatball mixture, roll into balls, and place on the baking sheet. (This makes about 40 small meatballs.) Bake for 15 minutes, remove from the oven, and set aside.

Meanwhile, in a large soup pot over medium heat, add the avocado oil. Sauté the celery, onion, bell pepper, and garlic for 5 minutes, or until the vegetables are soft.

Pour in the chicken stock, water, tomatoes (with juice), Italian seasoning, and sea salt. Bring to a boil, reduce to a low simmer, and cover. Allow the soup to simmer for 30 to 45 minutes.

Remove the lid and add the cooked meatballs, kale, and parsley. Cook for another 10 minutes, or until the meatballs are fully cooked through.

BUFFALO CHILI

SERVINGS: 6 TO 8
TIME: 1 HOUR, 20 MINUTES

2 pounds ground bison meat
1 large poblano pepper, diced
½ large onion, diced
3 garlic cloves, minced
1 (15-ounce) can diced fire-roasted tomatoes
1 (15-ounce) can tomato sauce
1 cup beef broth
¼ cup chili powder
1 tablespoon ground cumin
1 teaspoon sea salt
Diced avocado, grass-fed shredded cheese, and sour cream for garnish (optional)

In a large stockpot over medium heat, brown the bison meat.

Add the pepper, onion, and garlic. Stir well and cook for 10 minutes.

Stir in the tomatoes (with juice), tomato sauce, and broth. Add the chili powder, cumin, and sea salt.

Bring to a boil, stir well, reduce the heat to low, and cover. Allow to simmer for about 1 hour, stirring occasionally.

Serve with the toppings (if using).

SPAGHETTI AND MARINARA MEAT SAUCE

SERVINGS: 4
TIME: I HOUR, 10 MINUTES

I spaghetti squash
2 tablespoons coconut oil
I pound ground beef
½ cup diced bell pepper
2 garlic cloves, minced
½ cup diced onion
I zucchini, diced
I pint cherry tomatoes, sliced
I (29-ounce) canned tomato puree
I teaspoon sea salt
2 teaspoons dried basil
2 tablespoons apple cider vinegar

Preheat the oven to 400°F.

Slice the spaghetti squash in half lengthwise, scoop out the seeds, and rub the insides with I tablespoon of the coconut oil. Place the squash cut side down on a rimmed baking sheet and bake for 45 minutes to I hour, or until fork-tender.

In a large skillet over medium-high heat, brown the ground beef. Set the meat aside on a plate.

In the same skillet, add the remaining I tablespoon coconut oil and sauté the bell pepper, garlic, and onion for 5 minutes. Add the zucchini and cherry tomatoes and cook for 7 to 8 minutes, or until soft.

Add the tomato puree, sea salt, dried basil, and vinegar. Stir well, reduce the heat to low, and let simmer until the zucchini is done.

Once the squash is finished cooking, remove from the oven.

Add the meat to the tomato sauce and stir to combine.

Scrape the inside of the spaghetti squash with a fork and place the strands in a bowl. Top with the meat sauce and enjoy.

Make It Vegan

Omit the ground beef and top the dish with sliced avocado.

STEAK AND VEGGIE KEBABS

SERVINGS: 4
TIME: 40 MINUTES

MARINADE:

1/2 cup extra virgin olive oil

1/4 cup coconut aminos

1 tablespoon lemon juice

2 teaspoons Dijon mustard

1/2 teaspoon sea salt

1/4 teaspoon ground black pepper

KEBABS:

1 pound sirloin steak

2 large bell peppers

2 large zucchinis

1 large onion

2 tablespoons extra virgin olive oil, plus more for the grill

8 wooden skewers, soaked in water for 20 minutes

Sea salt, to taste

In a medium bowl, mix together the marinade ingredients.

Cut the steak into 1-inch pieces and place in a large resealable storage bag. Add the marinade to the meat and marinate in the refrigerator for at least 3 hours.

Cut the vegetables into large chunks of about equal size and place in a large bowl. Toss in the extra virgin olive oil.

Preheat a grill to 425°F and brush with olive oil.

Place the vegetables and marinated steak onto the soaked skewers, alternating steak and vegetables. Salt the steak and vegetables to taste and place on the grill. Turn every few minutes. Cook until the internal temperature of the steak registers 145°F and the veggies are cooked as desired, about 10 minutes.

Serve warm.

SALMON CAKES WITH GARLIC AIOLI

SERVINGS: 8
TIME: 15 MINUTES

SALMON CAKE:

2 (14.75-ounce) cans wild-caught salmon

1 tablespoon avocado oil mayonnaise

2 green onions, chopped

½ small bell pepper, diced

¼ cup finely diced fresh parsley or dill

¼ cup almond flour

2 eggs

Pinch of sea salt

2 tablespoons avocado oil

GARLIC AIOLI:

¼ cup avocado oil mayonnaise

½ tablespoon Dijon mustard

½ tablespoon lemon juice

1 garlic clove, minced

In a medium bowl, mix together all the salmon cake ingredients, except the oil.

With clean hands, form 8 round patties about ½ inch thick.

In a large skillet over medium-high heat, add the oil. Carefully place the patties in the pan.

Cook the patties for 4 minutes, then flip and cook for another 3 to 4 minutes.

In a small bowl, whisk together the aioli ingredients. Pour into small ramekins and serve with the patties.

Give It a Collagen Boost:

Add 1 scoop of collagen protein to the salmon mixture before forming the patties.

KETO BUFFALO CHICKEN WINGS

SERVINGS: 2–3

TIME: 1 HOUR, 10 MINUTES

12 chicken wing pieces, or 6 whole wings

1 tablespoon avocado oil

1 teaspoon sea salt

4 tablespoons grass-fed butter or ghee

¼ cup hot sauce of choice

1 garlic clove, minced, or 1 teaspoon garlic powder

Preheat the oven to 400°F.

In a bowl, toss the chicken wings in the avocado oil and sea salt. Set a wire rack on a rimmed baking sheet and arrange the chicken wings so they aren't touching.

Bake for 50 minutes, and then increase the oven temperature to 425°F and bake for another 15 minutes. Be sure the chicken is cooked through and the internal temperature reaches 165°F.

In a small saucepan over medium-low heat, place the butter or ghee, hot sauce, and minced or powdered garlic and heat until the butter has melted, stirring frequently.

Toss the chicken wings in the warm hot sauce and serve immediately.

CHICKEN PESTO

SERVINGS: 4

TIME: 30 MINUTES

2 tablespoons avocado oil

4 chicken breast cutlets*

¼ cup coconut flour

2 cups fresh basil leaves

¼ cup extra virgin olive oil

¼ cup pine nuts

1 teaspoon sea salt

1 garlic clove

2 tablespoons fresh Parmesan cheese (optional)

*Note: If you can't find cutlets, simply cut breasts in a butterfly manner.

In a large skillet over medium heat, add the oil.

Coat each chicken cutlet with the coconut flour and then place in the skillet. Allow to cook for 3 to 4 minutes on each side.

Meanwhile, make the pesto by adding the remaining ingredients to a food processor and pulsing until blended together.

When the chicken is almost done, pour the pesto over the chicken and allow everything to cook for a few more minutes, until the chicken is cooked through and the internal temperature reaches 165°F.

Give It a Collagen Boost

Add 1 scoop of collagen protein to the pesto while blending.

CASHEW CHICKEN LETTUCE CUPS

SERVINGS: 4

TIME: 25 MINUTES

6 tablespoons coconut aminos

3 tablespoons almond butter

2 tablespoons coconut vinegar*

1 tablespoon minced fresh ginger

1 garlic clove, minced

1 teaspoon sesame oil

1 tablespoon coconut oil

1 cup diced bell peppers

1 pound chicken, cut into small pieces

½ cup roughly chopped cashews, plus more for topping

4 leaves butter lettuce

In a small bowl, whisk together the coconut aminos, almond butter, vinegar, ginger, garlic, and sesame oil. Set the sauce aside.

In a large skillet over medium heat, add the coconut oil. Once the oil is melted, add the bell peppers and sauté for 5 minutes, or until soft.

Add the chicken and 3 tablespoons of the sauce to the skillet and cook for 10 minutes, or until the chicken is cooked through and the added sauce cooks out.

Note: 1 tablespoon white balsamic vinegar plus 1 tablespoon apple cider vinegar also works in place of coconut vinegar.

Once the chicken is cooked, toss in the chopped cashews.

Pour the remaining sauce over the chicken, veggies, and cashews and mix well.

Add about ½ cup of the mixture to each lettuce leaf cup. Top with more cashews, if desired, and serve.

Make It Vegan

Use extrafirm tofu in place of the chicken.

COCONUT CHICKEN TENDERS

SERVINGS: 2–3
TIME: 45 MINUTES

¼ cup coconut flour
1 teaspoon sea salt
¼ teaspoon ground black pepper
¼ teaspoon garlic powder
2 eggs, beaten
1 cup unsweetened shredded coconut
1 pound chicken tenderloins (or 3 breasts, sliced lengthwise into 3
    tenders each)
2 tablespoons coconut oil, melted

Preheat the oven to 400°F. Place a wire rack on a rimmed baking sheet lined with parchment paper and lightly brush or spray with melted coconut oil to prevent sticking.

Arrange the following ingredients in 3 medium bowls: (1) the coconut flour mixed with the sea salt, black pepper, and garlic powder; (2) the beaten eggs; (3) the shredded coconut.

Coat the tenderloins in the coconut flour mixture, shaking off any excess. Then dredge them in the eggs, and finally roll them in the shredded coconut.

Place the coated tenders on the wire rack. Avoid overcrowding.

Using a pastry brush, lightly brush the tenders with the melted coconut oil.

Bake the tenders for 24 minutes, flipping halfway through.

VEGETARIAN CEVICHE WITH MUSHROOMS

SERVINGS: 5 TO 7
TIME: 30 MINUTES

2 cups chopped mushrooms of choice
2 avocados, diced
3 Roma tomatoes, chopped
I green bell pepper, chopped
I jalapeño, stem removed and chopped
I red onion, chopped (optional)
Juice of 4 to 5 limes
½ cup chopped fresh cilantro
Almond flour tortillas

In a large mixing bowl, add all the ingredients except the tortillas and mix until well combined.

Cover and refrigerate for 30 minutes.

Serve in the almond flour tortillas.

THAI COCONUT CHICKEN SOUP

SERVINGS: 6 TO 8

TIME: I HOUR

3 lemongrass stalks

8 cups chicken bone broth

I inch ginger, chopped

3 chicken breasts

½ shallot, sliced into rounds

I red bell pepper, sliced

1½ cups chopped mushrooms

I tablespoon red chili paste

I (16-ounce) can full-fat coconut milk

Juice of ½ small lime

I cup chopped fresh cilantro

Crush the lemongrass stalks.

In a large pot over medium-low heat, combine the lemongrass, broth, and ginger. Steep for 25 minutes.

Remove the ginger and lemongrass bits.

Add the chicken, shallot, pepper, mushrooms, and chili paste and bring to a boil.

Simmer on low for 20 minutes, or until the chicken is cooked through and the vegetables are soft.

Remove from the heat and shred the chicken breasts. Add the coconut milk, lime juice, and cilantro. Serve warm.

CAULIFLOWER STEAK

SERVINGS: 3 TO 4
TIME: 45 MINUTES

1 large head of cauliflower, sliced lengthwise through the core into 4 steaks
2 tablespoons ghee or avocado oil
1/2 teaspoon garlic powder
1/2 teaspoon sea salt
1 teaspoon Italian herb seasoning
Juice of 1/2 lemon

Preheat the oven to 350°F.

Place the cauliflower slices on a rimmed baking sheet lined with parchment paper.

Drizzle with the ghee or avocado oil and top with the seasonings and lemon juice.

Bake for 30 to 45 minutes, or until tender.

LAMB BURGERS

SERVINGS: 8
TIME: 40 MINUTES

1/2 medium red onion, sliced
1 pound minced lean lamb
1 pound lean ground beef
2 ounces raw aged sharp cheddar, cut into 1/2-inch cubes
1/2 tablespoon sea salt
2 teaspoons garlic powder
1/4 teaspoon smoked paprika
1 teaspoon dried oregano
1/2 teaspoon coconut oil
Lettuce, for serving

Place the onion in the bowl of a food processor and pulse until finely chopped.

Transfer the onion to a large mixing bowl and add the lamb, ground beef, cheese, and spices, using your hands to combine all the ingredients. Form 8 patties.

Chill in the refrigerator for 15 to 20 minutes, or until firm.

In a large nonstick skillet over medium-high heat, melt the coconut oil. Fry the burgers for 7 to 8 minutes per side, or until firm to the touch and nicely browned.

Serve hot with your favorite toppings on a bed of lettuce or serve wrapped in lettuce.

SEARED GRASS-FED STEAK

SERVINGS: 2 TO 4

TIME: 1 HOUR

2 (6-ounce) grass-fed beefsteaks (your favorite cut), no more than
    1½ inches thick
1 tablespoon finely chopped fresh rosemary
½ teaspoon onion powder
½ teaspoon garlic powder, plus more, to taste, for the mushrooms
Sea salt and ground black pepper, to taste
2 tablespoons plus 2 teaspoons avocado oil
1 cup sliced mushrooms

Preheat the oven to 350°F.

Remove the steaks from the refrigerator and place them in a baking dish. Allow the steaks to come to room temperature, 20 to 30 minutes.

In a small bowl, combine the rosemary, onion powder, garlic powder, sea salt, and pepper.

Pat the steaks dry and sprinkle each side with the rosemary mixture. Place the baking dish in the oven and bake the steaks for 10 minutes, flipping halfway through. With 2 minutes remaining on the timer, heat a large skillet over medium-high heat.

Remove the steaks from the oven. Add 2 teaspoons of the avocado oil to the hot skillet and immediately add the steaks. Cook for 2 to 4 minutes on each side, to your desired doneness, and sprinkle with more sea salt and pepper. Remove the steaks from the skillet and allow them to rest for 5 to 8 minutes.

Meanwhile, in the same skillet over medium heat, add the remaining 2 tablespoons avocado oil. Add the mushrooms and season to taste with sea salt, pepper, and garlic powder. Sauté for about 5 minutes, or until lightly browned.

Serve the steaks topped with the sautéed mushrooms and enjoy.

SLOW COOKER BEEF AND BROCCOLI

SERVINGS: 2
TIME: 6 TO 8 HOURS

1/4 cup coconut aminos

2 tablespoons white wine

2 tablespoons apple cider vinegar

2 tablespoons ghee

1 tablespoon coconut oil

2 garlic cloves, chopped

1/2 teaspoon red pepper flakes

1 pound thin beef rib eye, sliced into strips

1 head broccoli, broken into pieces

1 tablespoon sesame seeds

In a slow cooker, add the coconut aminos, wine, vinegar, ghee, oil, garlic, and red pepper flakes. Stir well.

Add the beef and coat with the mixture.

Cover and cook on low for 6 to 8 hours.

Add the broccoli to the slow cooker 1 hour before serving.

Top with the sesame seeds and serve.

ZUCCHINI LASAGNA

SERVINGS: 6
TIME: 45 MINUTES

1 red onion, diced

4 garlic cloves, minced

2 tablespoons extra virgin olive oil

2½ pounds grass-fed ground beef

2 tablespoons chopped fresh oregano

2 tablespoons chopped fresh basil

½ teaspoon cayenne pepper

½ teaspoon sea salt

3 cups diced tomatoes

1 (6-ounce) can tomato paste

1 cup pitted black olives, sliced

6 zucchinis, thinly sliced (or 2 eggplants, thinly sliced)

1 cup shredded raw cheese or buffalo mozzarella

Preheat the oven to 350°F.

In a large pot over medium-low heat, sauté the onion and garlic in the olive oil for about 3 minutes.

Add the ground beef and brown it.

Add the oregano, basil, cayenne pepper, and sea salt. Stir well.

Mix in the diced tomatoes and tomato paste.

In a greased 9- x 13-inch baking dish, place a layer of sliced zucchini or eggplant, and then ladle on a thick layer (about half) of the meat mixture. Top with the sliced black olives.

Add another layer of sliced zucchini or eggplant, and then top with the remaining meat mixture.

Add the cheese on top.

Cover tightly with aluminum foil and bake for 30 minutes.

Make It Vegan

Omit the ground beef and use a dairy-free cheese.

KETO PIZZA CRUST

SERVINGS: 4 TO 6
TIME: I HOUR

4 medium zucchini
I cup plus 3 tablespoons arrowroot flour
½ cup coconut flour
3 eggs

Preheat the oven to 350°F.

Wash and grate the zucchini.

Squeeze the water out of the grated zucchini and place it in a medium bowl, discarding the zucchini juice.

Add the arrowroot flour, coconut flour, and eggs. Mix until well combined.

Line a 12-inch round pizza pan with parchment paper and place the batter on the paper. Use your fingers to press the batter into shape until it forms a thin, round pizza crust.

Bake for 40 to 45 minutes, flipping halfway through.

KETO FLORENTINE PIZZA

SERVINGS: 4 TO 6
TIME: I HOUR, 15 MINUTES

Keto Pizza Crust (recipe above)
2 cups fresh spinach
¼ cup fresh basil
¼ cup sun-dried tomatoes
¼ cup grated Pecorino Romano
¼ cup grated raw sheep's milk cheese
¼ cup crumbled goat cheese
¼ cup fresh buffalo mozzarella, sliced
4 eggs
Red pepper flakes, to taste
Ground black pepper, to taste
Dried oregano, to taste

Make the Keto Pizza Crust and leave the oven on.

When the crust is finished, scatter the spinach, basil, tomatoes, Pecorino Romano, sheep's milk cheese, goat cheese, and mozzarella on top.

Crack the eggs on top of the pizza.

Sprinkle with red pepper flakes, black pepper, and oregano, if desired.

Bake the pizza until the eggs are cooked to the desired doneness, 12 to 15 minutes.

SIDES

BAKED ZUCCHINI SLICES

SERVINGS: 4

TIME: 30 MINUTES

2 zucchinis
1 tablespoon avocado oil
1 teaspoon dried thyme
Sea salt and ground black pepper, to taste
⅓ cup grated Parmesan cheese (optional)

Preheat the oven to 400°F.

Slice the zucchini into ¼-inch slices.

In a medium bowl, toss the zucchini with the oil, thyme, sea salt, and pepper.

Arrange in a single layer on a rimmed baking sheet and top with the Parmesan cheese (if using).

Bake for 20 minutes. If desired, finish under the broiler for about 1 minute to brown the cheese.

Make It Vegan

Use a dairy-free cheese to top the zucchini instead of Parmesan, or simply omit to also make it Paleo-friendly.

CHEESY BROCCOLI

SERVINGS: 4
TIME: 30 MINUTES

1 pound broccoli florets (fresh or frozen)
4 tablespoons grass-fed butter, ghee, or coconut oil
1/2 teaspoon sea salt
1 cup shredded cheddar cheese
1/4 cup shredded fresh Parmesan cheese

Preheat the oven to 400°F.

In a large pot over medium-high heat, bring about 1 inch of water to a boil. Add the broccoli, cover, and cook for 5 minutes.

Drain the broccoli and add it to a medium greased casserole dish.

Add the butter and mix until evenly distributed. Top with the sea salt and cheese.

Bake for 20 minutes, or until the cheese begins to brown.

Make It Vegan

Use coconut oil and dairy-free cheese to make this both vegan and dairy-free.

SAUTÉED SPINACH

SERVINGS: 4
TIME: 12 MINUTES

2 tablespoons avocado oil
1 garlic clove, minced
12 ounces fresh baby spinach*
Juice of 1/2 lemon
Sea salt, to taste

In a large skillet over medium heat, add the oil and garlic.

*Note: This recipe also works with 1 pound of frozen spinach. Follow the directions on the bag of frozen spinach for stovetop cooking, then drain all excess liquid. Use as you would fresh spinach.

Sauté the garlic for 1 to 2 minutes, or until fragrant and slightly browned.

Add the spinach (it will fill the skillet entirely but will cook down) and coat with the oil and garlic mixture. Cover and allow to wilt for 5 minutes.

Remove the lid after 5 minutes and stir well.

Remove from the heat, toss with the lemon juice, and add the sea salt to taste.

CAULIFLOWER RICE WITH CILANTRO AND LIME

SERVINGS: 6 TO 8

TIME: 15 TO 20 MINUTES

2 tablespoons grass-fed butter

4 cups grated cauliflower

3 garlic cloves, minced

Juice of 1 lime

½ cup chopped fresh cilantro

Sea salt and ground black pepper, to taste

In a large pan, melt the butter over medium-high heat.

Add the cauliflower and minced garlic.

Cook the cauliflower, stirring occasionally, for 5 to 10 minutes and then remove from the heat.

Place the cauliflower mixture in a large mixing bowl, pour in the lime juice, and mix well.

Stir in the chopped cilantro.

Add the sea salt and pepper and serve immediately.

MASHED CAUL-TATOES

SERVINGS: 2 TO 4
TIME: 15 MINUTES

1 medium head cauliflower (about 1½ pounds), quartered
¼ cup grass-fed butter
¼ cup minced fresh chives
3 roasted garlic cloves, chopped
½ teaspoon sea salt
½ teaspoon ground black pepper

In a large pot filled halfway with water, boil the cauliflower for 7 to 10 minutes, or until tender.

Drain the cauliflower.

In a food processor, add the cauliflower, butter, chives, garlic, sea salt, and pepper.

Blend until smooth. Serve hot.

BUTTER-BAKED BRUSSELS SPROUTS

SERVINGS: 2 TO 4
TIME: 35 MINUTES

4 cups Brussels sprouts, halved
1 small red onion, cut into crescents
½ cup chopped walnuts
2 tablespoons grass-fed butter, melted
Sea salt and ground black pepper, to taste

Preheat the oven to 425°F.

In a medium bowl, combine the Brussels sprouts, onion, and walnuts. Mix in the butter until evenly distributed.

Sprinkle with the sea salt and pepper, and then spread the mixture out on a rimmed baking sheet lined with parchment paper.

Roast for 35 to 40 minutes, or until slightly browned.

CUCUMBER SALAD WITH TOMATO AND ONION

SERVINGS: 2 TO 4
TIME: 10 MINUTES

DRESSING:

2 to 3 tablespoons apple cider vinegar
2 to 3 tablespoons extra virgin olive oil
1/4 teaspoon sea salt
1/4 teaspoon ground black pepper

SALAD:

1 cucumber, quartered
12 Kumato tomatoes, halved
1/2 red onion, chopped
2 to 3 green onions, chopped
Chiffonade of 8 basil leaves

In a small bowl, mix together the dressing ingredients until well combined. Set aside.

In a medium bowl, combine the salad ingredients.

Drizzle the dressing onto the salad, mix together thoroughly, and serve.

STRAWBERRY SPINACH SALAD WITH POPPY SEED DRESSING

SERVINGS: 4 TO 6
TIME: 12 MINUTES

DRESSING:

1/2 cup extra virgin olive oil
2 tablespoons apple cider vinegar
1 1/2 tablespoons poppy seeds
1 tablespoon lemon juice

SALAD:

6 cups fresh spinach

2 cups chopped strawberries

1/2 red onion, diced

1 avocado, diced

1/4 to 1/2 cup goat's milk feta

1/4 cup sprouted almonds, chopped

In a small bowl, mix all the dressing ingredients until well combined. Set aside.

In a large bowl, combine all the salad ingredients.

Pour the dressing onto the salad and mix until well combined.

Refrigerate for 20 minutes and then serve.

Make It Vegan

Replace the feta with dairy-free cheese.

GRILLED ASPARAGUS

SERVINGS: 2 TO 3

TIME: 15 MINUTES

3 tablespoons coconut oil

1 bunch asparagus

5 garlic cloves, chopped

Sea salt, to taste

In a large skillet over medium-high heat, melt the coconut oil.

Add the remaining ingredients to the pan. Cover and cook for 10 minutes, stirring occasionally. Continue to cook until desired tenderness is achieved.

LOADED SPAGHETTI SQUASH

SERVINGS: 2 TO 4
TIME: 25 MINUTES

I spaghetti squash
Chiffonade of 10 basil leaves
I cup chopped sun-dried tomatoes
4 ounces sheep's milk feta, crumbled
2 tablespoons extra virgin olive oil
2 tablespoons balsamic vinegar
Sea salt and ground black pepper, to taste

Preheat the oven to 400°F.

Line a rimmed baking sheet with parchment paper.

Slice the spaghetti squash in half lengthwise, scoop out the seeds, and rub the insides with I tablespoon of the coconut oil. Place the squash cut side down on a rimmed baking sheet and bake for 45 minutes to I hour, or until fork-tender.

Scrape out the spaghetti squash into a large bowl.

Top the spaghetti squash with the basil, sun-dried tomatoes, and feta.

In a small bowl, whisk together the oil, vinegar, sea salt, and pepper. Pour over the spaghetti squash mixture and toss to distribute the dressing throughout.

Serve warm.

CAJUN COLLARD GREENS

SERVINGS: 6 TO 8
TIME: 6 TO 8 HOURS

8 cups chopped collard greens
8 ounces turkey bacon, chopped
3 cups chicken bone broth
2 tablespoons Dijon mustard
1 teaspoon garlic powder
1/4 teaspoon onion powder
1/2 teaspoon dried oregano
1/2 teaspoon dried thyme
1/2 teaspoon smoked paprika
1/4 teaspoon cayenne pepper
1 teaspoon sea salt
1 teaspoon ground black pepper

In a slow cooker, combine all the ingredients. Cover and cook on low for 6 to 8 hours.

SAUTÉED SUMMER VEGGIES

SERVINGS: 4
TIME: 15 MINUTES

1 tablespoon coconut oil
5 garlic cloves, sliced
2 yellow squash, halved lengthwise and sliced
1 zucchini, halved lengthwise and sliced
1/2 teaspoon sea salt
1/2 teaspoon ground black pepper
1 cup red grape tomatoes
2 tablespoons chopped fresh oregano

In a large skillet over medium-high heat, heat the oil.
Add the garlic and cook, stirring constantly, for about 30 seconds.

Add the yellow squash, zucchini, sea salt, and pepper. Stir and cook for about 3 minutes.

Stir in the tomatoes and continue cooking for 3 more minutes, or until the vegetables are tender.

Remove from the heat and stir in the oregano.

SAUERKRAUT

YIELD: ABOUT 1 GALLON

TIME: 30 MINUTES ACTIVE PREP; 4 WEEKS TOTAL

1 large head cabbage, shredded

3 tablespoons pickling salt

1 tablespoon caraway seeds

1 onion, quartered

In a large bowl, mix the cabbage with 2 tablespoons of the salt. Let stand for 10 minutes.

Massage the cabbage to release the juices for about 10 minutes.

Sprinkle the remaining 1 tablespoon salt and the caraway seeds onto the cabbage.

Pack the cabbage mixture in a large glass container that has a lid. Top with the onion, and place the lid on the container. Make sure the cabbage is completely submerged in the liquid.

Place the container on a plate and leave in a cool spot (unrefrigerated) for 2 weeks. Check the cabbage every other day to make sure it is submerged in the liquid. Skim off any film that forms on the surface of the fluid.

Let it stand for another 2 weeks, then store in an airtight container in the refrigerator for up to 6 months.

SAUCES, DIPS, AND DRESSINGS

TAHINI LEMON DRESSING

YIELD: 1¼ CUPS
TIME: 5 MINUTES

½ cup tahini
Juice of 1 large lemon
2 tablespoons extra virgin olive oil
1 teaspoon sea salt
1 teaspoon Dijon mustard
1 garlic clove, minced
½ cup water

In a small bowl, whisk together all the ingredients except the water. Gradually stir in the water until the dressing reaches the desired consistency.

CASHEW CAESAR DRESSING

YIELD: 1 CUP
TIME: 5 MINUTES

½ cup raw cashews, soaked in water for at least 6 hours and drained
Juice of ½ lemon
3 oil-packed anchovy fillets
2 teaspoons Dijon mustard
2 garlic cloves, minced
½ teaspoon sea salt
2 tablespoons extra virgin olive oil
⅓ cup water

In a high-speed blender, blend all the ingredients except the water. Gradually add the water until the dressing reaches the desired consistency.

Make It Vegan

Replace the anchovies with 2 teaspoons capers.

Give It a Collagen Boost

Add 1 scoop of collagen protein before blending.

CINNAMON NUT BUTTER

YIELD: 2 CUPS
TIME: 15 MINUTES

1½ cups dry-roasted unsalted almonds
1½ cups dry-roasted unsalted cashews
2 tablespoons nut oil (macadamia, almond, or cashew)
1 tablespoon ground cinnamon or pumpkin pie spice
¼ teaspoon sea salt
1 teaspoon pure vanilla extract

Combine all the ingredients in a high-speed blender.
Blend for 10 minutes or longer, until a creamy consistency forms.

Give It a Collagen Boost

Add 1 scoop of collagen protein before blending.

AVOCADO RANCH DRESSING

YIELD: 2 CUPS
TIME: 35 MINUTES

1 cup goat's milk kefir
2 tablespoons chopped scallions
2 teaspoons chopped fresh thyme
2 teaspoons chopped fresh parsley
1 teaspoon chopped fresh dill
2 teaspoons roasted garlic
¼ teaspoon onion powder
Sea salt and cracked black pepper, to taste
2 very ripe avocados

Combine all the ingredients in a food processor and process until well combined and creamy.

SUPER CILANTRO GUACAMOLE

SERVINGS: 4
TIME: 5 MINUTES

3 ripe avocados
¾ cup chopped fresh cilantro
½ heirloom tomato, chopped
½ medium red onion, chopped
I jalapeño, stem and seeds removed, chopped
Juice of I lime
I teaspoon garlic powder
I teaspoon ground cumin
I teaspoon smoked paprika

Place the avocados in a medium bowl and mash.

Add the remaining ingredients and continue to mash and stir until well combined.

Serve with a keto-friendly veggie, such as celery, bell pepper, or cucumber.

CAULIFLOWER HUMMUS

SERVINGS: 4
TIME: I HOUR

I medium head of cauliflower
4 tablespoons extra virgin olive oil, plus more for drizzling
½ cup tahini
2 large garlic cloves
⅓ cup lemon juice
I teaspoon sea salt
½ teaspoon ground black pepper
Chopped fresh parsley, to taste (optional)

Preheat the oven to 425°F, and line a rimmed baking sheet with parchment paper.

Remove the florets from the cauliflower and place in a large bowl. Add 2 tablespoons of the olive oil, toss to coat, then pour the florets onto the baking sheet. Roast for 20 minutes.

In a food processor, combine the roasted cauliflower, tahini, remaining 2 tablespoons olive oil, garlic, lemon juice, sea salt, and pepper and process until smooth.

Pour the hummus into an airtight container and place in the refrigerator until cold.

Serve in a bowl and top with the parsley and a drizzle of olive oil (if using).

HOLLANDAISE SAUCE

YIELD: ¼ cup

TIME: 5 TO 7 MINUTES

2 tablespoons grass-fed butter or ghee, melted

1 egg yolk

¼ teaspoon Dijon mustard

1 tablespoon lemon juice

¼ teaspoon sea salt

1½ teaspoons water

In a high-speed blender, blend all the ingredients until well combined.

SNACKS

CHIA PUDDING

SERVINGS: 1
TIME: 2 HOURS, 5 MINUTES

¼ cup full-fat canned coconut milk
¼ cup unsweetened almond milk
2 tablespoons chia seeds
1 tablespoon hempseeds
½ cup berries of choice
1 scoop vanilla collagen protein

In a small bowl, stir together the coconut milk, almond milk, and chia seeds. Chill in the refrigerator for at least 2 hours, or overnight.

Once chilled, stir the pudding well. Mix in the hempseeds, berries, and collagen protein. Serve and enjoy.

KETO FAT BOMBS

SERVINGS: 12
TIME: 1 HOUR, 10 MINUTES

8 tablespoons (1 stick) grass-fed butter
½ cup crunchy almond butter
1 teaspoon pure vanilla extract
½ teaspoon ground cinnamon

In a small saucepan over medium-low heat, melt the butter and almond butter. Remove from the heat.

Add the vanilla and cinnamon, stirring until well combined.

Line a muffin pan with liners and equally distribute the mixture into the pan.

Freeze for 30 minutes to 1 hour.

KETO BREAD

SERVINGS: 20 (1 SLICE PER SERVING)
TIME: 40 MINUTES

6 eggs, separated
¼ teaspoon cream of tartar
1½ cups almond flour
3 to 4 tablespoons grass-fed butter, melted
¾ teaspoon baking soda*
1 tablespoon apple cider vinegar*

Preheat the oven to 375°F.

In a medium bowl, combine the egg whites and cream of tartar. Using a hand mixer, whip the eggs until soft peaks form.

In a food processor, combine the egg yolks and remaining ingredients and blend until well incorporated.

Transfer the mix to a medium bowl and gently fold in the egg white mixture.

Grease an 8- x 4-inch loaf pan and pour in the batter.

Bake for 30 minutes.

*Note: You can substitute 1 tablespoon baking powder for the ¾ teaspoon
    baking soda and 1 tablespoon apple cider vinegar, if desired.

KETO CUPS

SERVINGS: 24
TIME: 1 HOUR, 10 MINUTES

½ cup coconut oil
½ cup almond butter
15 to 20 drops liquid stevia
2 teaspoons pure vanilla extract
2 tablespoons cacao powder or unsweetened cocoa powder

In a small saucepan over medium-low heat, melt the coconut oil and almond butter. Remove from the heat.

Add the stevia, vanilla, and cacao powder, stirring until well combined.

Line a mini-muffin pan with liners and equally distribute the mixture into the pan.

Freeze for 30 minutes to 1 hour.

KALE CHIPS

SERVINGS: 2 TO 4
TIME: 15 MINUTES

1 bunch kale
2 tablespoons grapeseed or avocado oil
1 tablespoon lemon juice
1/4 teaspoon sea salt

Preheat the oven to 350°F.

Chop the kale into 1/2-inch pieces.

Combine all the ingredients in a large bowl and massage the oil, lemon juice, and sea salt into the kale using your hands.

Place the kale on a rimmed baking sheet lined with parchment paper and bake for 12 minutes.

Remove from the oven and serve.

KETO COOKIE DOUGH BARS

SERVINGS: 6
TIME: 30 MINUTES

2/3 cup cashew or almond butter
1/2 cup unsweetened chocolate chips
2 scoops vanilla bone broth protein
3 tablespoons coconut cream
1 egg

Preheat the oven to 325°F.

In a food processor, add all the ingredients and blend well. Stop, scrape down the sides, and blend again.

On a rimmed baking sheet lined with parchment paper, form the dough into a rectangle, about ¼ inch thick.

Bake for 20 minutes.

Remove and allow to cool completely.

Cut into six bars.

Make It Vegan

Omit the bone broth protein and the egg. Add ½ teaspoon pure vanilla extract. Bake at 250°F.

COLLAGEN-BOOSTING BLUEBERRY MUFFINS

SERVINGS: 12
TIME: 35 MINUTES

2 cups almond flour
½ cup coconut flour
1½ teaspoons baking powder
¼ teaspoon sea salt
2 scoops keto collagen powder
⅓ cup canned coconut milk
3 eggs
¼ cup monk-fruit sweetener
3 tablespoons coconut oil, melted
¾ cup blueberries

Preheat the oven to 350°F.

In a large bowl, mix together the flours, baking powder, sea salt, and collagen powder. Set aside.

In a medium bowl, whisk together the coconut milk, eggs, monk-fruit sweetener, and coconut oil.

Slowly add the milk mixture to the flour mixture, mixing well.

Fold in the blueberries and scoop the mixture into a lined or sprayed muffin tin. Bake for 20 minutes.

Make It Vegan

Replace the eggs with 3 tablespoons flaxseed powder plus ½ cup water, and omit the keto collagen powder.

GRANOLA

SERVINGS: 4 TO 6
TIME: 35 MINUTES

½ cup unsweetened shredded coconut

I cup raw almonds, slivered or sliced

I cup raw walnuts or cashews

I cup raw pecans

½ cup raw pumpkin seeds

¼ cup hempseeds

I cup cacao nibs

I teaspoon ground cinnamon or pumpkin pie spice

¼ teaspoon sea salt

¼ cup coconut oil, melted

2 tablespoons maple-flavored monk-fruit sweetener

Preheat the oven to 325°F.

In a large bowl, mix together all the ingredients except the coconut oil and monk-fruit sweetener.

In a large saucepan over medium-low heat, warm and stir the coconut oil and monk-fruit sweetener. Add the other ingredients and mix well.

Line a rimmed baking sheet with parchment paper and spread the mixture onto it. Bake for 20 minutes. Remove and toss around with a spatula. Bake for another 5 minutes, or until golden brown.

KETO DEVILED EGGS

SERVINGS: 12 (2 DEVILED EGGS PER SERVING)

TIME: 18 MINUTES

12 eggs
1/4 cup avocado oil mayonnaise
1 tablespoon Dijon mustard
1 teaspoon apple cider vinegar
1 teaspoon dill pickle juice
1 teaspoon sea salt
1/2 teaspoon ground black pepper
Paprika, to taste

In a large pot over medium-high heat, place the eggs in enough water to cover and bring to a boil. Cover the pot and turn off the heat. Let sit for 8 minutes.

After 8 minutes, remove the eggs with a large slotted spoon and submerge them in a large bowl filled with ice water.

When the eggs have cooled, remove the shells and slice in half lengthwise. Carefully remove the yolks and add them to a medium-size mixing bowl.

Whisk the remaining ingredients except the paprika into the yolks until blended.

Spoon or pipe the yolk mixture into the hollow of each egg half. Sprinkle with paprika and enjoy.

DESSERTS

For additional delicious dessert recipes, go to www.draxe.com/keto
-diet-desserts.

CHOCOLATE AVOCADO MOUSSE

SERVINGS: 3 TO 4
TIME: 10 MINUTES

1 teaspoon pure vanilla extract
1½ cups mashed avocado (2 to 3 avocados)
2 scoops chocolate keto protein powder (or 2 scoops collagen
    protein plus 1 tablespoon MCT oil) or chocolate bone broth
    protein
¼ cup cacao powder
½ cup water

In a food processor, combine the vanilla, avocado, keto protein
powder, and cacao powder. Process until creamy, stopping to scrape
down the sides of the bowl with a spatula, if needed.
    Add the water and process until smooth.
    Serve at room temperature or chilled. Store in a sealed container in
the refrigerator for up to 3 days or in the freezer for up to 2 weeks.

PEPPERMINT PATTIES

SERVINGS: 10
TIME: 30 MINUTES

½ cup plus 2 tablespoons coconut oil, softened
1 tablespoon coconut cream
½ teaspoon liquid stevia
1 teaspoon peppermint extract
¾ cup unsweetened chocolate chips

In a small bowl, mix together ½ cup of the coconut oil, the coconut cream, stevia, and peppermint extract. Using a tablespoon, spoon the mixture onto a baking sheet or plate lined with parchment paper and form into 10 flattened patties.

Place in the freezer for 10 minutes to allow to harden.

In a small saucepan over low heat, melt the chocolate chips and the remaining 2 tablespoons coconut oil together. Using a fork, dip the frozen peppermint patties into the chocolate mixture and place back on the parchment paper.

Place back in the freezer until the chocolate has hardened, about 10 minutes.

LEMON BARS

SERVINGS: 16
TIME: 50 MINUTES

CRUST:

6 tablespoons ghee or grass-fed butter
2 cups almond flour
2 tablespoons stevia powder (about 10 packets)
1 tablespoon grated lemon zest

FILLING:

½ cup ghee or grass-fed butter, melted
2 scoops collagen protein
3 eggs
½ cup lemon juice
2 tablespoons stevia powder (about 10 packets)
4 drops liquid stevia
2 tablespoons grated lemon zest
Pinch of sea salt

Preheat the oven to 350°F. Line an 8- x 8-inch baking pan with parchment paper.

In a medium bowl, combine all the ingredients for the crust and press into the bottom of the pan. Bake for 10 minutes.

Cut into 16 squares.

To make the filling, in a medium bowl, whisk together the melted ghee and collagen protein.

Add the remaining filling ingredients to the butter mixture. Pour over the baked crust.

Bake for another 20 minutes. Remove and allow to cool, then place in the refrigerator for at least 2 hours, or until fully set.

KETO PEANUT BUTTER COOKIES

SERVINGS: 12

TIME: 22 MINUTES

1 cup all-natural peanut butter

$\frac{1}{3}$ cup monk-fruit sweetener

$\frac{2}{3}$ cup almond flour

1 egg

1 scoop keto collagen powder

$\frac{1}{4}$ teaspoon sea salt

Preheat the oven to 350°F.

In a medium bowl, combine all the ingredients and mix well.

Using a tablespoon, scoop the batter onto a rimmed baking sheet lined with parchment paper, about 2 tablespoons per ball, placed about 2 inches apart. Using a fork, press the balls down in a crosshatch pattern.

Bake for 12 minutes.

Make It Vegan

Replace the egg with 1 tablespoon flaxseed powder plus 3 tablespoons water. Omit the keto collagen powder, and add $\frac{1}{4}$ teaspoon pure vanilla extract.

KETO CHOCOLATE CHIP COOKIES

SERVINGS: 24

TIME: 22 MINUTES

2 cups almond flour

1 scoop collagen protein

1/2 teaspoon baking powder

1/4 teaspoon sea salt

1/2 cup coconut oil, melted

1/2 cup monk-fruit sweetener

1 teaspoon pure vanilla extract

2 eggs

1/2 cup unsweetened chocolate chips

Preheat the oven to 350°F.

In a large bowl, mix together the almond flour, collagen protein, baking powder, and sea salt. Set aside.

In a separate bowl, mix together the coconut oil, monk-fruit sweetener, vanilla, and eggs.

Incorporate the coconut oil mixture into the flour mixture until a thick batter forms. Stir in the chocolate chips.

Scoop and roll the batter into 24 equal-size balls and gently press down with the back of a spoon or your fingertips. Place 2 inches apart on a rimmed baking sheet lined with parchment paper. Bake for 10 to 12 minutes.

KETO FUDGE

SERVINGS: 9

TIME: 35 MINUTES

1 cup coconut butter

1 cup almond butter

2 tablespoons cacao powder or unsweetened cocoa powder

1 tablespoon chocolate bone broth protein

1/2 cup melted coconut oil, plus more if needed

1 teaspoon liquid stevia

1/4 teaspoon sea salt

In a food processor, combine all the ingredients and blend until the mixture is smooth, adding more melted coconut oil as needed to achieve desired texture.

Pour the mixture into an 8- x 8-inch baking dish lined with parchment paper.

Freeze for at least 30 minutes, or until ready to serve. Cut into thirds one way and again into thirds the other way.

TOASTED COCONUT MACAROONS

SERVINGS: 10 TO 12

TIME: 45 MINUTES

2 cups unsweetened shredded coconut

2 egg whites

¼ cup monk-fruit sweetener

½ teaspoon baking powder

½ teaspoon pure vanilla or almond extract

Pinch of sea salt

¼ cup 80% or more dark chocolate, melted (optional)

Preheat the oven to 350°F.

Place the shredded coconut on a rimmed baking sheet and toast for 5 minutes. Remove and allow to cool. Reduce the heat to 325°F.

In a medium bowl, whip the egg whites with a handheld blender until soft peaks form. Slowly add the monk-fruit sweetener, baking powder, vanilla, and sea salt while whisking gently.

Gently fold in the toasted coconut until fully incorporated.

Scoop into 10 to 12 equal-size balls and place on a rimmed baking sheet lined with parchment paper.

Bake for 10 minutes. Reduce the heat to 300°F and bake for another 20 minutes.

Remove and allow to cool. Once cooled, dip the bottoms into the melted dark chocolate (if using) and return to the parchment paper. Once the chocolate has hardened, enjoy.

KETO BROWNIES

SERVINGS: 16
TIME: 50 MINUTES

1/2 cup almond flour

1/4 cup cacao powder or unsweetened cocoa powder

1/2 teaspoon sea salt

1/2 teaspoon baking powder

2 ounces unsweetened dark chocolate

1/2 cup coconut oil

1/2 cup monk-fruit sweetener

3 eggs, at room temperature

1/2 teaspoon pure vanilla extract

Preheat the oven to 350°F. Line an 8- x 8-inch baking pan with parchment paper.

In a medium bowl, mix the flour, cocoa powder, sea salt, and baking powder.

Using a double boiler (or a microwave), melt the dark chocolate and coconut oil together and stir until smooth. (If using the microwave, heat at 30-second intervals, stirring between intervals.)

In a separate bowl, beat the sweetener, eggs, and vanilla vigorously.

Add the chocolate mixture and continue to mix.

Fold in the flour mixture and mix until a batter forms.

Pour into the lined baking pan and bake for 20 minutes, or until a toothpick inserted into the center comes out clean. Cut into 16 squares.

Make It Vegan

Replace the eggs with 3 tablespoons flaxseed powder plus 1/2 cup water.

Give It a Collagen Boost

Add 2 scoops collagen protein to the flour mixture.

KETO CHEESECAKE

SERVINGS: 10 TO 12
TIME: 1 HOUR, 25 MINUTES

CRUST:

1½ cups almond flour

1 packet stevia powder

5 tablespoons cultured butter, melted

1 teaspoon pure vanilla extract

FILLING:

24 ounces cream cheese, softened

1 tablespoon stevia powder (about 5 packets)

½ cup coconut cream

2 eggs

1 teaspoon grated lemon zest

SIMPLE BLUEBERRY TOPPING (OPTIONAL):

1 cup blueberries

5 to 6 drops liquid stevia

Preheat the oven to 350°F.

In a small bowl, mix together the crust ingredients. Press into the bottom of a 9-inch springform pan and bake for 10 minutes. Remove and allow to cool.

Reduce the oven temperature to 300°F.

To make the filling, in a medium bowl, mix together the cream cheese and stevia. Slowly add the coconut cream until fully incorporated. Scrape down the sides of the bowl.

Add the eggs, one at a time, while whisking. Add the lemon zest.

Pour the cream cheese mixture into the springform pan on top of the crust.

Bake for 1 hour. Remove from the oven and allow to cool completely. Cool in the fridge for 3 hours (or overnight). Do not try to remove the cake from the pan until it has been chilled.

To make the optional topping, in a small saucepan over low heat, heat the blueberries and stevia together, and slightly mash the blueberries with a fork. Serve on top of the cheesecake.

Make It Vegan

FOR THE CRUST:

Replace the butter with coconut oil.

FOR THE FILLING:

16 ounces cashew-based vegan cream cheese

1 cup unsweetened coconut yogurt

1 teaspoon grated lemon zest

1 teaspoon lemon juice

1 tablespoon stevia powder (about 5 packets)

2 tablespoons coconut oil, melted

In a medium bowl, whisk together all the filling ingredients until incorporated and creamy. Pour on top of the baked crust and freeze for about 1 hour. Once firm, it is ready to enjoy.

KETO CHOCOLATE FROSTY

SERVINGS: 1

TIME: 35 MINUTES

1 cup canned coconut milk

2 tablespoons cacao powder or unsweetened cocoa powder

1 tablespoon almond butter

1 teaspoon pure vanilla extract

1 tablespoon stevia powder (about 5 packets)

In a medium bowl, whisk together all the ingredients with an electric hand mixer, stand mixer, or a hand whisk for 30 seconds, or until the ingredients are fully incorporated, thick, and creamy.

Freeze for 30 minutes, or until a frosty consistency forms. Whisk again for smoothness and enjoy.

Give It a Collagen Boost

Add 1 scoop of keto collagen powder.

KETO FUDGESICLES

SERVINGS: 6 TO 8
TIME: 3 HOURS, 10 MINUTES

3 cups full-fat coconut milk
2 scoops chocolate bone broth protein
Pinch of sea salt

In a saucepan over medium-low heat, whisk together all the ingredients until warmed throughout and completely incorporated and creamy.

Pour the mixture into ice-pop molds and place in the freezer for 3 hours, or until fully frozen.

CHAPTER 18

Keto Diet Shopping List

Fats and Oils (organic, high-quality)

Animal fats (tallow and
    schmaltz)
Avocado
Avocado oil
Cacao nibs (unsweetened)
Chia seed oil
Coconut cream (the cream
    skimmed off the top of
    canned organic coconut
    milk)
Coconut oil
Dark chocolate (80% and up)

Extra virgin olive oil
Flaxseed oil
Ghee (clarified butter)
Grapeseed oil
Grass-fed butter
Macadamia nut oil
MCT oil
Olives
Red palm oil
Sesame oil
Unsweetened chocolate chips

Proteins

Red Meat (organic, grass-fed)

Beef
Bison
Buffalo
Elk

Goat (chevon)
Lamb
Venison

Poultry (organic, free-range)

Chicken

Duck

Organ meats (liver, kidney,
and heart)

Pheasant

Turkey

Turkey bacon

Eggs (cage-free)

Eggs, chicken

Eggs, duck

Seafood (wild-caught)

Anchovy fillets

Bass

Cod

Grouper

Haddock

Halibut

Mackerel

Mahimahi

Ocean perch

Salmon

Sardines

Snapper

Tilapia

Tuna

Dairy (full-fat, organic, grass-fed)

Cottage cheese

Cream cheese

Yogurt

Goat's milk cheese

Goat's milk cottage cheese

Goat's milk kefir

Hard cheeses (cheddar, jack,
colby, Parmesan, chèvre,
Manchego)

Sheep's milk feta

Sour cream

Protein powders

Bone broth protein

Collagen protein

Keto collagen powder

Keto protein powder

Vegetables (organic)

Anise/fennel

Artichokes

Arugula

Asparagus

Beet greens

Bok choy

Broccoli

Brussels sprouts

Cabbage

Carrots

Cauliflower

Celery

Chard

Chives

Collard greens

Cucumbers

Dill pickles (no sugar added)

Garlic

Green beans

Greens

Kale

Kohlrabi

Leeks

Lemongrass

Lettuce (all types)

Mushrooms (all types)

Okra

Olives

Onions/scallions/shallots

Peppers (bell, jalapeño, poblano)

Radishes

Rhubarb

Snow/sugar snap peas

Spinach

Sprouts

Squash

Tomatoes

Tomatoes, canned (roasted; with green chilies; diced)

Tomato paste, canned

Tomato puree, canned

Tomato sauce, canned

Turnips

Zucchini

Fruits (organic)

Avocado

Blackberries

Blueberries

Grapefruit

Lemon

Lime

Raspberries

Strawberries

Nuts and Seeds

Almonds

Almond butter

Almond flour

Almond flour tortillas

Almond meal

Brazil nuts

Cashews

Chia seeds

Coconut

Coconut butter

Coconut flour

Flaxseeds

Hazelnuts

Hempseeds

Macadamia nuts
Peanut butter
Pecans
Pine nuts
Pistachios
Poppy seeds

Pumpkin seeds/pepitas
Sesame seeds
Sunflower seeds
Tahini
Walnuts

Sweeteners

Monk fruit
Stevia

Fermented Foods

Fermented assorted veggies
Kimchi

Raw apple cider vinegar
Sauerkraut

Seasonings, Herbs, and Baking Needs

Baking powder
Baking soda
Basil
Bay leaves
Black pepper
Cacao powder
Cayenne pepper
Chili powder
Cilantro
Cinnamon
Cocoa powder
Coriander
Cream of tartar
Cumin
Dill
Garlic powder
Ginger (fresh and ground)
Goji berry powder
Horseradish

Italian herb seasoning
Mint
Mustard powder
Onion powder
Oregano
Paprika/smoked paprika
Parsley
Peppermint extract
Pink Himalayan salt
Pumpkin pie spice
Pure vanilla extract
Red chili paste
Red pepper flakes
Rosemary
Sage
Sea salt
Thyme
Turmeric

Condiments

Apple cider vinegar

Balsamic vinegar

Coconut aminos

Coconut vinegar

Hot sauce

Ketchup (low sugar)

Mayonnaise
(avocado oil–based)

Mustard (yellow and Dijon)

White wine

Beverages

Almond milk (unsweetened)

Coconut milk

Coffee (preferably organic)

Purified water

Sparkling mineral water

Tea (herbal, unsweetened,
matcha, green, oolong,
Eleotin, and yerba maté)

Resources

3-Day Keto Collagen Cleanse Plan: www.draxe.com/keto-diet-collagen
Bonus Keto Desserts: www.draxe.com/keto-diet-desserts
Dr. Axe's Keto360 Program, with recipes and supplement plan: www.draxe.com/keto-diet-keto-360
Keto Cycling Menu Plan: www.draxe.com/keto-diet-cyclingplan
My Mom's Keto Cancer Plan: www.draxe.com/keto-diet-cancerplan
Quick-Start Guide with All the Keto Diet Essentials: www.draxe.com/keto-diet-kickstarter
Top Keto Diet Foods Everyone Should Eat: www.draxe.com/keto-diet-food-lists
Top Keto Supplements and How to Use Them: www.draxe.com/keto-diet-supplements
Top Metabolism Boosters: www.draxe.com/keto-diet-metabolism

To stay up-to-date on the latest keto diet and health news, be sure to follow me and my wife, Chelsea, on social media:

Facebook: www.facebook.com/DrJoshAxe/
YouTube: Dr. Josh Axe channel (www.youtube.com/channel/UCgtp61tf9tYF7nGgIQ94LQ)
Instagram: drjoshaxe and drchelseaaxe

Acknowledgments

I want to thank the brilliant Ginny Graves for helping me create this book. Also, my sincere thanks to the entire Little, Brown Spark team, especially Tracy Behar and Peggy Freudenthal, for their fantastic insights, editing, and vision for what this book could be. I am grateful to my literary agent, Bonnie Solow, who is the best in the business and always goes above and beyond. I also want to express my heartfelt gratitude to Jordan Rubin, my closest friend and business partner, for inspiring me to write this book. And to my entire team at Ancient Nutrition: Thank you for all your hard work and sincere commitment to improving the health of our country and our world. Finally, my deepest appreciation to those of you who follow me on social media and visit my website—and who bought this book. Here's to you for investing in your well-being and taking your health to the next level!

Big Blessings!
Dr. Josh Axe

Notes

CHAPTER 1 *The Diet That Works When Nothing Else Will*

1. John S. O'Brien and E. Lois Sampson, "Lipid Composition of the Normal Human Brain: Gray Matter, White Matter and Myelin," *Journal of Lipid Research* 6 (October 1965): 537–544.
2. Priya Sumithran, Luke A. Prendergast, Elizabeth Delbridge, et al., "Long-Term Persistence of Hormonal Adaptations to Weight Loss," *New England Journal of Medicine* 365 (October 27, 2011): 1597–1604.
3. Cara B. Ebbeling, Janis F. Swain, Henry A. Feldman, et al., "Effects of Dietary Composition on Energy Expenditure during Weight-Loss Maintenance," *Journal of the American Medical Association* 307 (June 27, 2012): 2627–2634.
4. P. Sumithran, L. A. Prendergast, E. Delbridge, et al., "Ketosis and Appetite-Mediating Nutrients and Hormones after Weight Loss," *European Journal of Clinical Nutrition* 67 (July 2013): 759–764.
5. Philip B. Maffetone and Paul B. Laursen, "The Prevalence of Overfat Adults and Children in the US," *Frontiers in Public Health* 5 (November 2017).
6. Raj Padwal, William D. Leslie, Lisa M. Lix, and Sumit R. Majumdar, "Relationship among Body Fat Percentage, Body Mass Index and All-Cause Mortality: A Cohort Study," *Annals of Internal Medicine* 164 (April 2016): 532–541.
7. Centers for Disease Control and Prevention, "Trends in Intake of Energy and Macronutrients in Adults from 1999–2000 through 2007–2008," NCHS Data Brief no. 49, November 2010.
8. Anahad O'Connor, "Rethinking Weight Loss and the Reasons We're 'Always Hungry,'" *New York Times*, January 7, 2016, https://well.blogs.nytimes.com/2016/01/07/rethinking-weight-loss-and-the-reasons-were-always-hungry/.
9. Iris Shai, Dan Schwarzfuchs, Yaakov Henkin, et al., "Weight Loss with a Low-Carbohydrate, Mediterranean, or Low-Fat Diet," *New England Journal of Medicine* 359 (July 17, 2008): 229–241.

CHAPTER 2 *The Keto Diet Advantage*

1. Centers for Disease Control and Prevention, "New CDC Report: More than 100 Million Americans Have Diabetes or Prediabetes," CDC Newsroom Releases, July 18, 2017.

2. Centers for Disease Control and Prevention, "Long-Term Trends in Diabetes," April 2017, https://www.cdc.gov/diabetes/statistics/slides/long_term_trends.pdf.

3. Eric C. Westman, William S. Yancy Jr., John C. Mavropoulos, Megan Marquart, and Jennifer R. McDuffie, "The Effect of a Low-Carbohydrate, Ketogenic Diet versus a Low-Glycemic Control in Type 2 Diabetes Mellitus," *Nutrition & Metabolism* 5 (December 19, 2008).

4. A. Paoli, A. Rubini, J. S. Volek, and K. A. Grimaldi, "Beyond Weight Loss: A Review of the Therapeutic Uses of Very-Low-Carbohydrate (Ketogenic) Diets," *European Journal of Clinical Nutrition* 67 (2013): 789–796.

5. N. B. Bueno, I. S. Vieira de Melo, S. Lima de Oliveira, and T. da Rocha Ataide, "Very-Low-Carbohydrate Ketogenic Diet v. Low-Fat Diet for Long-Term Weight Loss: A Meta-Analysis of Randomized Controlled Trials," *British Journal of Nutrition* 110 (October 2013): 1178–1187.

6. Hussein M. Dashti, Thazhumpal C. Mathew, Talib Hussein, et al., "Long-Term Effects of a Ketogenic Diet in Obese Patients," *Experimental & Clinical Cardiology* 9 (2004): 200–205.

7. J. W. Wheless, "History of the Ketogenic Diet," *Epilepsia* 49 (November 2008): 3–5.

8. Samuel Livingston, *Comprehensive Management of Epilepsy in Infancy, Childhood and Adolescence* (Springfield, IL: Charles C. Thomas Publisher, 1972), 378–405.

9. Paoli et al., "Beyond Weight Loss."

10. Matthew K. Taylor, Debra K. Sullivan, Jonathan D. Mahnken, Jeffrey M. Burns, and Russell H. Swerdlow, "Feasibility and Efficacy Data from a Ketogenic Diet Intervention in Alzheimer's Disease," *Alzheimer's & Dementia* 4 (2018): 28–36; Robert Krikorian, Marcelle D. Shidler, Krista Dangelo, Sarah C. Couch, Stephen C. Benoit, and Deborah J. Clegg, "Dietary Ketosis Enhances Memory in Mild Cognitive Impairment," *Neurobiology of Aging* 33 (2012): 19–27; M. Ota, J. Matsuo, I. Ishida, et al., "Effect of a Ketogenic Meal on Cognitive Function in Elderly Adults: Potential for Cognitive Enhancement," *Psychopharmacology* 233 (2016): 3797–3802.

11. T. B. Vanitallie, C. Nonas, A. Di Rocco, K. Boyar, K. Hyams, and S. B. Heymsfield, "Treatment of Parkinson Disease with Diet-Induced Hyperketonemia: A Feasibility Study," *Neurology* 64 (February 22, 2005): 728–730.

12. Eleonora Napoli, Nadia Dueñas, and Cecilia Giulivi, "Potential Therapeutic Use of the Ketogenic Diet in Autism Spectrum Disorders," *Frontiers in Pediatrics* 2 (June 30, 2014).

13. M. J. Tisdale, R. A. Brennan, and K. C. Fearon, "Reduction of Weight Loss and Tumour Size in a Cachexia Model by a High Fat Diet," *British Journal of Cancer* 56 (1987): 39–43.

14. Bryan G. Allen, Sudershan K. Bhatia, Carryn M. Anderson, et al., "Ketogenic Diets as an Adjuvant Cancer Therapy: History and Potential Mechanism," *Redox Biology* 2 (2014): 963–970.

15. Richard Weindruch and Rajindar S. Sohal, "Caloric Intake and Aging," *New England Journal of Medicine* 337 (1997): 986–994.

16. J. Traba, M. Kwarteng-Siaw, T. C. Okoli, et al., "Fasting and Refeeding Differentially Regulate NLRP3 Inflammasome Activation in Human Subjects," *Journal of Clinical Investigation* 125 (November 2015): 4592–4600.

17. J. C. Newman, A. J. Covarrubias, M. Zhao, et al., "Ketogenic Diet Reduces Midlife Mortality and Improves Memory in Aging Mice," *Cell Metabolism* 26 (September 2017): 547–557.

18. Mahshid Dehghan, Andrew Mente, Xiaohe Zhang, et al., "Associations of Fats and Carbohydrate Intake with Cardiovascular Disease and Mortality in 18 Countries from Five Continents (PURE): A Prospective Cohort Study," *Lancet* 390 (November 2017): 2050–2062.

CHAPTER 3 *How to Kick-Start Ketosis*

1. Nicole M. Aven, P. Rada, and B. G. Hoebel, "Evidence for Sugar Addiction: Behavioral and Neurochemical Effects of Intermittent, Excessive Sugar Intake," *Neuroscience and Biobehavioral Reviews* 32 (2008): 20–39.

2. Wendy S. White, Y. Zhou, A. Crane, P. Dixon, F. Quadt, and L. M. Flendrig, "Modeling the Dose Effects of Soybean Oil in Salad Dressing on Carotenoid and Fat-Soluble Vitamin Bioavailability in Salad Vegetables," *American Journal of Clinical Nutrition* 106 (August 2017): 1041–1051.

3. M. P. St.-Onge, R. Ross, W. D. Parsons, and P. J. Jones, "Medium-Chain Triglycerides Increase Energy Expenditure and Decrease Adiposity in Overweight Men," *Obesity Research* 11 (March 2003): 395–402.

4. H. Singh, T. Kaur, S. Manchanda, and G. Kaur, "Intermittent Fasting Combined with Supplementation with Ayurvedic Herbs Reduces Anxiety in Middle Aged Female Rats by Anti-Inflammatory Pathways," *Biogerontology* 4 (August 2017): 601–614.

5. T. Anwer, M. Sharma, K. K. Pillai, and M. Iqbal, "Effect of Withania somnifera on Insulin Sensitivity in Non-Insulin-Dependent Diabetes Mellitus Rats," *Basic & Clinical Pharmacology & Toxicology* 102 (June 2008): 498–503.

6. A. Chopra, P. Lavin, B. Patwardhan, and D. Chitre, "A 32-Week Randomized, Placebo-Controlled Clinical Evaluation of RA-11, an Ayurvedic Drug, on Osteoarthritis of the Knees," *Journal of Clinical Rheumatology* 10 (October 2004): 236–245.

7. Dushani L. Palliyaguru, S. V. Singh, and T. W. Kensler, "Withania somnifera: From Prevention to Treatment of Cancer," *Molecular Nutrition & Food Research* 60 (June 2016): 1342–1353.

8. Jonathon L. Reay, A. B. Scholey, and D. O. Kennedy, "Panax ginseng (G115) Improves Aspects of Working Memory Performance and Subjective Ratings of Calmness in Healthy Young Adults," *Human Psychopharmacology: Clinical & Experimental* 25 (August 2010): 462–471.

9. C. W. Davy, C. L. Yang, S. C. Chik, et al., "Bioactivity-Guided Identification and Cell Signaling Technology to Delineate the Immunomodulatory Effects of Panax ginseng on Human Promonocytic U937 Cells," *Journal of Translational Medicine* 7 (May 2009).

10. Zhipeng Li and Geun Eog Ji, "Ginseng and Obesity," *Journal of Ginseng Research* 42 (January 2018): 1–8.

11. Xiangli Cui, Y. Jin, D. Poudyal, et al., "Mechanistic Insight into the Ability of American Ginseng to Suppress Cancer Associated with Colitis," *Carcinogenesis* 31 (August 2010): 1734–1741.

12. H. J. Park, H. Y. Kim, K. H. Yoon, K. S. Kim, and I. Shim, "The Effects of Astragalus membranaceus on Repeated Restraint Stress-Induced Biochemical Behavioral Responses," *Korean Journal of Physiology Pharmacology* 13 (August 2009): 315–319.

13. Q. Qin, J. Niu, Z. Wang, W. Xu, Z. Qiao, and Y. Gu, "Astragalus membranaceus Extract Activates Immune Response in Macrophages via Heparanase," *Molecules* 17 (June 2012): 7232–7240.

14. Liangliang Zhou, L. Chen, J. Wang, and Y. Deng, "Astragalus Polysaccharide Improves Cardiac Function in Doxorubicin-Induced Cardiomyopathy through ROS-p38 Signaling," *International Journal of Clinical and Experimental Medicine* 8 (November 2015): 21839–21848.

15. Bin Yang, B. Xiao, and T. Sun, "Antitumor and Immunomodulatory Activity of *Astragalus membranaceus* Polysaccharides in H22 Tumor-Bearing Mice," *International Journal of Biological Macromolecules* (November 2013): 287–290.

16. E. A. Al-Dujaili, C. J. Kenyon, M. R. Nicol, and J. I. Mason, "Liquorice and Glycyrrhetinic Acid Increase DHEA and Deoxycorticosterone Levels in Vivo and in Vitro by Inhibiting Adrenal SULT2A1 Activity," *Molecular and Cellular Endocrinology* 336 (April 2011): 102–109.

17. Qing-Chun Huang, M. J. Wang, X. M. Chen, et al., "Can Active Components of Licorice, Glycyrrhizin and Glycyrrhetinic Acid Lick Rheumatoid Arthritis?" *Oncotarget* 7 (January 2016): 1193–1202.

18. E. M. Olsson, B. von Schéele, and A. G. Panossian, "A Randomised, Double-Blind, Placebo-Controlled, Parallel-Group Study of the Standardised Extract shr-5 of the Roots of Rhodiola rosea in the Treatment of Subjects with Stress-Related Fatigue," *Planta Medica* 75 (February 2009): 105–112.

19. A. Bystritsky, L. Kerwin, and J. D. Feusner, "A Pilot Study of Rhodiola rosea (Rhodax) for Generalized Anxiety Disorder," *Journal of Alternative and Complementary Medicine* 14 (March 2008): 175–180.

20. Jessica L. Verpeut, A. L. Walters, and N. T. Bello, "Citrus aurantium and Rhodiola rosea in Combination Reduce Visceral White Adipose Tissue and Increase Hypothalamic Norepinephrine in a Rat Model of Diet-Induced Obesity," *Nutrition Research* 33 (June 2013): 503–512.

21. Paola Rossi, D. Buonocore, E. Altobelli, et al., "Improving Training Condition Assessment in Endurance Cyclists: Effects of *Ganoderma lucidum* and *Ophiocordyceps sinensis* Dietary Supplementation," *Evidence-Based Complementary and Alternative Medicine* (April 2014).

22. E. A. Murphy, J. M. Davis, and M. D. Carmichael, "Immune Modulating Effects of Beta-Glucan," *Current Opinion in Clinical Nutrition & Metabolic Care* 13 (November 2010): 656–661.

23. C. Vandenberghe, V. St-Pierre, A. Courchesne-Loyer, M. Hennebelle, C. A. Castellano, and S. C. Cunnane, "Caffeine Intake Increases Plasma Ketones: An Acute Metabolic Study in Humans," *Canadian Journal of Physiology and Pharmacology* 95 (April 2017): 455–458.

CHAPTER 4 *A User's Guide to the Keto Diet*

1. Hedy Kober et al., study completed and in review.

2. Mary Enig, "Fat and Cholesterol in Human Milk," Weston A. Price Foundation, December 31, 2001, https://www.westonaprice.org/health-topics/childrens-health/fat-and-cholesterol-in-human-milk/.

3. M. A. Reger, S. T. Henderson, C. Hale, et al., "Effects of Beta-Hydroxybutyrate on Cognition in Memory-Impaired Adults," *Neurobiology of Aging* 25 (March 2004): 311–314.

4. K. Yamagishi, H. Iso, H. Yatsuya, et al., "Dietary Intake of Saturated Fatty Acids and Mortality from Cardiovascular Disease in Japanese: The Japan Collaborative Cohort Study for Evaluation of Cancer Risk (JACC) Study," *American Journal of Clinical Nutrition* 92 (October 2010): 759–765.

5. R. P. Mensink and M. B. Katan, "Effect of Dietary Fatty Acids on Serum Lipids and Lipoproteins: A Meta-Analysis of 27 Trials," *Arteriosclerosis and Thrombosis* 12 (August 1992): 911–919.

6. D. F. Hebeisen, F. Hoeflin, H. P. Reusch, E. Junker, and B. H. Lauterburg, "Increased Concentrations of Omega-3 Fatty Acids in Milk and Platelet Rich Plasma of Grass-Fed Cows," *International Journal of Vitamin and Nutrition Research* 63 (1993): 229–233.

7. Cynthia Daley, Amber Abbott, Patrick S. Doyle, Glenn A. Nader, and Stephanie Larson, "A Review of Fatty Acid Profiles and Antioxidant Content in Grass-Fed and Grain-Fed Beef," *Nutrition Journal* 10 (March 2010): 1–9.

8. Chenxi Qin, J. Lv, Y. Guo, et al., "Associations of Egg Consumption with Cardiovascular Disease in a Cohort Study of 0.5 Million Chinese Adults," *Heart* (May 2018).

9. Almudena Sánchez-Villegas, L. Verberne, J. De Irala, et al., "Dietary Fat Intake and the Risk of Depression: The SUN Project," *PLOS One* 6 (January 2011).

10. Mohammed Y. Yakoob, P. Shi, W. C. Willett, et al., "Circulating Biomarkers of Dairy Fat and Risk of Incident Diabetes Mellitus among Men and Women in the United States in Two Large Prospective Cohorts," *Circulation* 133 (March 2016): 1645–1654.

11. S. Rautiainen, L. Wang, I. M. Lee, J. E. Manson, J. E. Buring, and H. D. Sesso, "Dairy Consumption in Association with Weight Change and Risk of Becoming Overweight or Obese in Middle-Aged and Older Women: A Prospective Cohort Study," *American Journal of Clinical Nutrition* 103 (April 2016): 979–988.

12. B. Smith, "Organic Foods vs. Supermarket Foods: Element Levels," *Journal of Applied Nutrition* (1993).

13. S. Padrangi and L. F. LaBorde, "Retention of Folate, Carotenoids and Other Quality Characteristics in Commercially Packaged Fresh Spinach," *Journal of Food Science* (May 2006).

14. Joy C. Rickman, Diane M. Barrett, and Christine M. Bruhn, "Nutritional Comparison of Fresh, Frozen and Canned Fruits and Vegetables. Part 1. Vitamins C and B and Phenolic Compounds," *Journal of the Science of Food and Agriculture* 87 (2007): 930–944.

15. R. A. Hites, J. A. Foran, D. O. Carpenter, M. C. Hamilton, B. A. Knuth, and S. J. Schwager, "Global Assessment of Organic Contaminants in Farmed Salmon," *Science* 303 (January 2004): 226–229.

CHAPTER 5 *Super Keto Supplements*

1. D. R. Davis, M. D. Epp, and H. D. Riordan, "Changes in USDA Food Composition Data for 43 Garden Crops, 1950 to 1999," *Journal of the American College of Nutrition* 23 (December 2004): 669–682.

2. Brianna J. Stubbs, P. J. Cox, R. D. Evans, M. Cyranka, K. Clarke, and H. de Wet, "A Ketone Ester Drink Lowers Human Ghrelin and Appetite," *Obesity* 26 (February 2018): 269–273.

3. D. Choudhary, S. Bhattacharyya, and S. Bose, "Efficacy and Safety of Ashwagandha (Withania somnifera L. Dunal) Root Extract in Improving Memory and Cognitive Functions," *Journal of Dietary Supplements* 14 (November 2017): 599–612.

4. Mayo Clinic, "Healthy Lifestyle: Nutrition and Healthy Eating, Expert Answers," February 21, 2018, https://www.mayoclinic.org/healthy-lifestyle/nutrition-and-healthy-eating/expert-answers/functional-foods/faq-20057816.

5. Y. Takada, A. Bhardwaj, P. Potdar, and B. B. Aggarwal, "Nonsteroidal Anti-inflammatory Agents Differ in Their Ability to Suppress NF-kappaB Activation, Inhibition of Expression of Cyclooxygenase-2 and Cyclin D1, and Abrogation of Tumor Cell Proliferation," *Oncogene* 9 (December 2004): 9247–9258.

6. Cancer Research UK, "Turmeric," last reviewed August 6, 2015, https://www.cancerresearchuk.org/about-cancer/cancer-in-general/treatment/complementary-alternative-therapies/individual-therapies/turmeric.

7. B. Shan, Y. Z. Cai, M. Sun, and H. Corke, "Antioxidant Capacity of 26 Spice Extracts and Characterization of Their Phenolic Constituents," *Journal of Agricultural and Food Chemistry* 53 (October 2005): 7749–7759.

CHAPTER 6 *Keto Lifestyle Tactics*

1. Essential Oils Academy, "History of Essential Oils," https://essentialoilsacademy.com/history/.

2. Elizabeth Steels, A. Rao, and L. Vitetta, "Physiological Aspects of Male Libido Enhanced by Standardized *Trigonell foenum-graecum* Extract and Mineral Formulation," *Phytotherapy Research* 25 (September 2011): 1294–1300.

3. M. Khrosravi Samani, H. Mahmoodian, A. Moghadamnia, A. Poorsattar Bejeh Mir, and M. Chitsazan, "The Effect of Frankincense in the Treatment of Moderate Plaque-Induced Gingivitis: A Double Blinded Randomized Clinical Trial," *DARU Journal of Pharmaceutical Sciences* 19 (2011): 288–294.

4. S. Kasper, "An Orally Administered Lavandula Oil Preparation (Silexan) for Anxiety Disorder and Related Conditions: An Evidence Based Review," *International Journal of Psychiatry in Clinical Practice* (November 2013): 15–22.

5. B. Uehleke, S. Schaper, A. Dienel, S. Schlaefke, and R. Stange, "Phase II Trial on the Effects of Silexan in Patients with Neurasthenia, Post-Traumatic Stress Disorder or Somatization Disorder," *Phytomedicine* 19 (June 2012): 665–671.

6. G. Cappello, M. Spezzaferro, L. Grossi, L. Manzoli, and L. Marzio, "Peppermint Oil (Mintoil) in the Treatment of Irritable Bowel Syndrome: A Prospective Double Blind Placebo-Controlled Randomized Trial," *Digestive and Liver Disease* 39 (June 2007): 530–536.

7. Mark Moss and Lorraine Oliver, "Plasma 1,8-Cineole Correlates with Cognitive Performance Following Exposure to Rosemary Essential Oil Aroma," *Therapeutic Advances in Psychopharmacology* 2 (June 2012): 103–113.

8. S. Enshaieh, A. Jooya, A. H. Siadat, and F. Iraji, "The Efficacy of 5% Topical Tea Tree Oil Gel in Mild to Moderate Acne Vulgaris: A Randomized Double-Blind Placebo-Controlled Study," *Indian Journal of Dermatology, Venereology and Leprology* 73 (January–February 2007): 22–25.

9. American Institute of Stress, "America's #1 Health Problem," https://www.stress.org/americas-1-health-problem/.

10. Veronique A. Taylor, V. Daneault, J. Grant, et al., "Impact of Meditation Training on the Default Mode Network during a Restful State," *Social Cognitive and Affective Neuroscience* 8 (January 2013): 4–14.

11. Mei-Kei Leung, W. K. W. Lau, C. C. H. Chan, S. S. Y. Wong, A. L. C. Fung, and T. M. C. Lee, "Meditation-Induced Neuroplastic Changes in Amygdala Activity during Negative Affective Processing," *Social Neuroscience* 13 (April 2017): 277–288.

12. Britta K. Holzel et al., "Mindfulness Practice Leads to Increases in Regional Brain Gray Matter Density," *Psychiatry Research* 191 (January 2011): 36–43.

13. M. Jackowska, J. Brown, A. Ronaldson, and A. Steptoe, "The Impact of a Brief Gratitude Intervention on Subjective Well-Being, Biology and Sleep," *Journal of Health Psychology* 21 (October 2016): 2207–2217.

14. Laura Redwine, B. L. Henry, M. A. Pung, et al., "A Pilot Randomized Study of a Gratitude Journaling Intervention on HRV and Inflammatory Biomarkers in Stage B Heart Failure Patients," *Psychosomatic Medicine* 78 (July–August 2016): 667–676.

15. Debra Umberson and Jennifer Kara Montez, "Social Relationships and Health: A Flashpoint for Health Policy," *Journal of Health and Social Behavior* 51 (2010): S54–S66.

16. B. J. Park, Y. Tsunetsugu, T. Kasetani, T. Kagawa, and Y. Miyazaki, "The Physiological Effects of Shinrin-yoku (Taking in the Forest Atmosphere or Forest Bathing): Evidence from Field Experiments in 24 Forests across Japan," *Environmental Health and Preventive Medicine* 15 (January 2010): 18–26.

17. Jeffrey M. Jones, "In U.S., 40% Get Less Than Recommended Amount of Sleep," December 19, 2013, Gallup, https://news.gallup.com/poll/166553/less-recommended-amount-sleep.aspx.

18. Shahrad Teheri, L. Lin, D. Austin, T. Young, and E. Mignot, "Short Sleep Duration Is Associated with Reduced Leptin, Elevated Ghrelin, and Increased Body Mass Index," *PLOS Medicine* 1 (December 2004).

19. Deloitte, "2016 Global Mobile Consumer Survey: US Edition," Deloitte Development, 2016, p. 4.

20. Thomas Weaver, "Bad Mood? Get Moving," University of Vermont, November 3, 2009, http://www.uvm.edu/it/?Page=news&storyID=10098&category=ucommall.

21. C. D. Reimer, G. Knapp, and A. K. Reimers, "Does Physical Activity Increase Life Expectancy? A Review of the Literature," *Journal of Aging Research* 11 (July 2012).

22. H. Arem, S. C. Moore, A. Patel, et al., "Leisure Time Physical Activity and Mortality: A Detailed Pooled Analysis of the Dose-Response Relationship," *JAMA Internal Medicine* 175 (June 2015): 959–967.

CHAPTER 7 *Keto Metabolism Makeover*

1. A. Paoli, A. Rubini, J. S. Volek, and K. A. Grimaldi, "Beyond Weight Loss: A Review of the Therapeutic Uses of Very-Low-Carbohydrate (Ketogenic) Diets," *European Journal of Clinical Nutrition* 67 (2013): 789–796.

2. Jennifer Abbasi, "Interest in the Ketogenic Diet Grows for Weight Loss and Type 2 Diabetes," *Journal of the American Medical Association* 319 (January 16, 2018): 215–217.

3. N. B. Bueno, I. S. Vieira de Melo, S. Lima de Oliveira, and T. da Rocha Ataide, "Very Low Carbohydrate Ketogenic Diet v Low-Fat Diet for Long-Term Weight Loss: A Meta-Analysis of Randomised Controlled Trials," *British Journal of Nutrition* 110 (October 2013): 1178–1187.

4. Madeline K. Gibas and Kelly J. Gibas, "Induced and Controlled Dietary Ketosis as a Regulator of Obesity and Metabolic Syndrome Pathologies," *Diabetes & Metabolic Syndrome* (November 2017).

5. Amy Miskimon Goss, Barbara A Gower, Taraneh Soleymani, Mariah Stewart, and Kevin Fontaine, "Effects of an Egg-Based, Carbohydrate-Restricted Diet on Body Composition, Fat Distribution, and Metabolic Health in Older Adults with Obesity: Preliminary Results from a Randomized Controlled Trial," *FASEB Journal* (April 2017).

6. Sarah J. Hallberg, A. L. McKenzie, P. T. Williams, et al., "Effectiveness and Safety of a Novel Care Model for the Management of Type 2 Diabetes at 1 Year: An Open-Label, Non-Randomized, Controlled Study," *Diabetes Therapy* 9 (April 2018): 583–612.

7. Jeff S. Volek, S. D. Phinney, C. E. Forsythe, et al., "Carbohydrate Restriction Has a More Favorable Impact on the Metabolic Syndrome than a Low Fat Diet," *Lipids* 44 (April 2009): 297–309.

8. P. Sumithran, L. A. Prendergast, E. Delbridge, et al., "Ketosis and Appetite-Mediating Nutrients and Hormones after Weight Loss," *European Journal of Clinical Nutrition* 67 (July 2013): 759–764.

9. Antonio Paoli, G. Bosco, E. M. Camporesi, and D. Mangar, "Ketosis, Ketogenic Diet and Food Intake Control: A Complex Relationship," *Frontiers in Psychology* 6 (February 2015).

10. Priya Sumithran, Luke A. Prendergast, Elizabeth Delbridge, "Long-Term Persistence of Hormonal Adaptations to Weight Loss," *New England Journal of Medicine* 365 (October 2011): 1597–1604.

11. Liu Lin Thio, "Hypothalamic Hormones and Metabolism," *Epilepsy Research* 100 (July 2012): 245–251.

12. Pam Harrison, "Almost Half the US Population Has Diabetes or Its Precursor," Medscape, July 19, 2017, https://www.medscape.com/viewarticle/883132.

13. Thomas Reinehr, "Type 2 Diabetes Mellitus in Children and Adolescents," *World Journal of Diabetes* 4 (December 2013): 270–281.

14. Elizabeth J. Mayer-Davis, Jean M. Lawrence, Dana Dabelea, et al., "Incidence Trends of Type 1 and Type 2 Diabetes among Youths, 2002–2012," *New England Journal of Medicine* 376 (April 2017): 1419–1429.

15. I. Partsalaki, A. Karvela, and B. Spiliotis, "Metabolic Impact of a Ketogenic Diet Compared to a Hypocaloric Diet in Obese Children and Adolescents," *Journal of Pediatric Endocrinology and Metabolism* 25 (2012): 697–704.

16. University of California San Francisco, Sugar Science, "How Much Is Too Much?" http://sugarscience.ucsf.edu/the-growing-concern-of-overconsumption.html#.W3sglJNKhEI.

17. Sanjay Basu, Paula Yoffe, Nancy Hills, and Robert H. Lustig, "The Relationship of Sugar to Population-Level Diabetes Prevalence: An Economic Analysis of Repeated Cross-Sectional Data," *PLOS One* 8 (February 2013).

18. Alison B. Evert, Jackie L. Boucher, Marjorie Cypress, et al., "Nutrition Therapy Recommendations for the Management of Adults with Diabetes," *Diabetes Care* 36 (November 2013).

19. H. M. Dashti, Thazhumpal C. Mathew, Talib Hussein, et al., "Long-Term Effects of a Ketogenic Diet in Obese Patients," *Experimental & Clinical Cardiology* 9 (Fall 2004): 200–205.

20. M. P. St-Onge and P. J. Jones, "Greater Rise in Fat Oxidation with Medium-Chain Triglyceride Consumption Relative to Long-Chain Triglyceride Is Associated with Lower Initial Body Weight and Greater Loss of Subcutaneous Adipose Tissue," *International Journal of Obesity and Related Metabolic Disorders* 27 (December 2003): 1565–1571.

21. R. A. Anderson, N. Cheng, N. A. Bryden, et al., "Elevated Intakes of Supplemental Chromium Improve Glucose and Insulin Variables in Individuals with Type 2 Diabetes," *Diabetes* 46 (November 1997): 1786–1791.

22. T. Kim, J. Davis, A. J. Zhang, X. He, and S. T. Mathews, "Curcumin Activates AMPK and Suppresses Gluconeogenic Gene Expression in Hepatoma Cells," *Biochemical and Biophysical Research Communications* 388 (October 2009): 377–382.

23. Nafiseh Khandouzi, F. Shidfar, A. Rajab, T. Rahideh, P. Hosseini, and M. Mir Taheri, "The Effects of Ginger on Fasting Blood Sugar, Hemoglobin A1c, Apolipoprotein B, Apolipoprotein A-I and Malondialdehyde in Type 2 Diabetic Patients," *Iranian Journal of Pharmaceutical Research* 14 (Winter 2015): 131–140.

24. L. Nogara, N. Naber, E. Pate, M. Canton, C. Reggiani, and R. Cooke, "Piperine's Mitigation of Obesity and Diabetes Can Be Explained by Its Up-Regulation of the Metabolic Rate of Resting Muscle," *Proceedings of the National Academy of Sciences* 113 (November 2016): 13009–13014.

CHAPTER 8 *Your Brain on Keto*

1. Maciej Gasior, Michael A. Rogawski, and Adam L. Hartman, "Neuroprotective and Disease-Modifying Effects of the Ketogenic Diet," *Behavioral Pharmacology* 17 (September 2006): 431–439.

2. Alzheimer's Association, "2018 Alzheimer's Disease Facts and Figures," https://www.alz.org/media/Documents/alzheimers-facts-and-figures-infographic.pdf.

3. Ibid.

4. World Health Organization, "Dementia: Key Facts," http://www.who.int/news-room/fact-sheets/detail/dementia.

5. Fanfan Zheng, L. Yan, Z. Yang, B. Zhong, W. Xie, "HbA1c, Diabetes and Cognitive Decline: The English Longitudinal Study of Aging," *Diabetologia* 61 (April 2018): 839–848.

6. Yang An, V. R. Varma, S. Varma, et al., "Evidence for Brain Glucose Dysregulation in Alzheimer's Disease," *Alzheimer's & Dementia* 14 (March 2018): 318–329.

7. Ingrid Van der Auwera, Stefaan Wera, Fred Van Leuven, and Samuel T. Henderson, "A Ketogenic Diet Reduces Amyloid Beta 40 and 42 in a Mouse Model of Alzheimer's Disease," *Nutrition & Metabolism* 2 (October 2005).

8. Matthew K. Taylor et al., "Feasibility and Efficacy Data from a Ketogenic Diet Intervention in Alzheimer's Disease," *Alzheimer's & Dementia: Translation Research & Clinical Interventions* 4 (2018): 28–36.

9. Rosebud O. Roberts, L. A. Roberts, Y. E. Geda, et al., "Relative Intake of Macronutrients Impacts Risk of Mild Cognitive Impairment or Dementia," *Journal of Alzheimer's Disease* 32 (January 2012): 329–339.

10. Steven C. Vlad et al., "Protective Effects of NSAIDs on the Development of Alzheimer Disease," *Neurology* 70 (May 2008): 1672–1677.

11. Markus Bock, Andreas Michalsen, and Friedemann Paul, "Ketogenic Diet and Prolonged Fasting Improve Health-Related Quality of Life and Lipid Profiles in Multiple

Sclerosis—A Randomized Controlled Trial" (Conference Paper, ECTRIMS 2015, Barcelona, October 2015).

12. T. E. Cullingford, "The Ketogenic Diet; Fatty Acids, Fatty Acid-Activated Receptors and Neurological Disorders," *Prostaglandins, Leukotrines and Essential Fatty Acids* 70 (March 2004): 253–264.

13. Mithu Storoni and Gordon T. Plant, "The Therapeutic Potential of the Ketogenic Diet in Treating Progressive Multiple Sclerosis," *Multiple Sclerosis International* (December 2015).

14. T. B. VanItallie, C. Nonas, A. Di Rocco, K. Boyar, K. Hyams, and S. B. Heymsfield, "Treatment of Parkinson Disease with Diet-Induced Hyperketonemia: A Feasibility Study," *Neurology* 64 (February 2005): 728–730.

15. O. El-Rashidy, F. El-Baz, Y. El-Gendy, R. Khalaf, D. Reda, and K. Saad, "Ketogenic Diet versus Gluten Free Casein Free Diet in Autistic Children: A Case-Control Study," *Metabolic Brain Disease* 32 (December 2017): 1935–1941.

16. E. C. Bostrok, Kenneth C. Kirkby, and Bruce V. M. Taylor, "The Current Status of the Ketogenic Diet in Psychiatry," *Frontiers in Psychiatry* 8 (March 2017).

17. C. Di Lorenzo, G. Coppola, G. Sirianni, et al., "Migraine Improvement during Short Lasting Ketogenesis: A Proof-of-Concept Study," *European Journal of Neurology* 22 (January 2015): 170–177.

18. Cherubino Di Lorenzo, Gianluca Coppola, Davide Di Lenola, et al., "Efficacy of Modified Atkins Ketogenic Diet in Chronic Cluster Headache: An Open-Label, Single-Arm Clinical Trial," *Frontiers in Neurology* 9 (February 2018).

19. Justin Sonnenburg and Erica Sonnenburg, "Gut Feelings—the 'Second Brain' in Our Gastrointestinal Systems," *Scientific American*, May 1, 2015, https://www.scientificamerican .com/article/gut-feelings-the-second-brain-in-our-gastrointestinal-systems -excerpt/.

20. Virginia Chaidez, Robin L. Hansen, and Irva Hertz-Picciotto, "Gastrointestinal Problems in Children with Autism, Developmental Delays or Typical Development," *Journal of Autism and Developmental Disorders* 44 (May 2014): 1117–1127.

21. D. Liu, Z. Wang, Z. Gao, et al., "Effects of Curcumin on Learning and Memory Deficits, BDNF, and ERK Protein Expression in Rats Exposed to Chronic Unpredictable Stress," *Behavioural Brain Research* 271 (September 2014): 116–121.

22. J. Sanmukhani, V. Satodia, J. Trivedi, et al., "Efficacy and Safety of Curcumin in Major Depressive Disorder: A Randomized Controlled Trial," *Phytotherapy Research* 28 (April 2014): 579–585.

23. David Kennedy, E. L. Wightman, J. L. Reay, et al., "Effects of Resveratrol on Cerebral Blood Flow Variables and Cognitive Performance in Humans: A Double-Blind, Placebo-Controlled, Crossover Investigation," *American Journal of Clinical Nutrition* 91 (June 2010): 1590–1597.

24. Esther M. Blessing, M. M. Steenkamp, J. Manzanares, and C. R. Marmar, "Cannabidiol as a Potential Treatment for Anxiety Disorders," *Neurotherapeutics* 12 (October 2015): 825–836.

25. S. Jazayeri, M. Tehrani-Doost, S. A. Keshavarz, et al., "Comparison of Therapeutic Effects of Omega-3 Fatty Acid Eicosapentaenoic Acid and Fluoxetine, Separately and in Combination, in Major Depressive Disorder," *New Zealand Journal of Psychiatry* 42 (July 2009): 192–198.

26. M. Friedman, "Chemistry, Nutrition, and Health-Promoting Properties of Hericium erinaceus (Lion's Mane) Mushroom Fruiting Bodies and Mycelia and Their Bioactive Compounds," *Journal of Agricultural and Food Chemistry* 19 (August 2015): 7108–7123.

27. Federico Brandalise, V. Cesaroni, A. Gregori, et al., "Dietary Supplementation of Hericium erinaceus Increases Mossy Fiber-CA3 Hippocampal Neurotransmission and Recognition Memory in Wild-Type Mice," *Evidence Based Complementary and Alternative Medicine* (2017).

28. K. Mori, S. Inatomi, K. Ouchi, Y. Azumi, and T. Tuchida, "Improving Effects of the Mushroom Yamabushitake (Hericium erinaceus) on Mild Cognitive Impairment: A Double-Blind Placebo-Controlled Trial," *Phytotherapy Research* 23 (March 2009): 367–372.

29. M. Moss, J. Cook, K. Wesnes, and P. Duckett, "Aromas of Rosemary and Lavender Essential Oils Differentially Affect Cognition and Mood in Healthy Adults," *International Journal of Neuroscience* 113 (January 2003): 15–38.

30. A. Cieza, P. Maier, and E. Pöppel, "Effects of Ginkgo Biloba on Mental Functioning in Healthy Volunteers," *Archives of Medical Research* 34 (September–October 2003): 373–381.

31. Georgia Ede, "Ketogenic Diets for Psychiatric Disorders: A New 2017 Review," *Psychology Today*, June 30, 2017, https://www.psychologytoday.com/us/blog/diagnosis-diet/201706/ketogenic-diets-psychiatric-disorders-new-2017-review.

CHAPTER 9 *Ketosis Is a Hero for Hormones*

1. Centers for Disease Control and Prevention, "PCOS and Diabetes, Heart Disease, Stroke," last updated March 14, 2018, https://www.cdc.gov/diabetes/library/spotlights/pcos.html.

2. John C. Mavropoulos, William S. Yancy, Juanita Hepburn, and Eric C Westman, "The Effects of a Low-Carbohydrate, Ketogenic Diet on the Polycystic Ovary Syndrome: A Pilot Study," *Nutrition & Metabolism* 2 (December 2005).

3. K. Yank, Liuting Zeng, Tingting Bao, and Jinwen Ge, "Effectiveness of Omega-3 Fatty Acid for Polycystic Ovary Syndrome: A Systematic Review and Meta-Analysis," *Reproductive Biology and Endocrinology* 16 (March 2018).

4. S. Kalgaonkar, R. U. Almario, D. Gurusinghe, et al., "Differential Effects of Walnuts vs. Almonds on Improving Metabolic and Endocrine Parameters in PCOS," *European Journal of Clinical Nutrition* 65 (March 2011): 386–393.

5. Debra A. Nowak, D. C. Snyder, A. J. Brown, and W. Demark-Wahnefried, "The Effect of Flaxseed Supplementation on Hormone Levels Associated with Polycystic Ovary Syndrome: A Case Study," *Current Topics in Nutraceutical Research* 5 (2007): 177–181.

6. Ming-Wei Lin and Meng-Hsing Wu, "The Role of Vitamin D in Polycystic Ovary Syndrome," *Indian Journal of Medical Research* 142 (September 2015): 238–240.

7. Melanie McGrice and Judi Porter, "The Effect of Low Carbohydrate Diets on Fertility Hormones and Outcomes in Overweight and Obese Women: A Systematic Review," *Nutrients* 9 (February 2017).

8. Hagai Levine, N. Jørgensen, A. Martino-Andrade, et al., "Temporal Trends in Sperm Count: A Systematic Review and Meta-Regression Analysis," *Human Reproduction Update* 23 (November 2017): 646–659.

9. Nancy A. Melville, "Carb Intake, Sperm Count Association Explored," Medscape, October 23, 2012, https://www.medscape.com/viewarticle/773202.

10. Jorge E. Chavarro, J. W. Rich-Edwards, B. A. Rosner, and W. C. Willett, "A Prospective Study of Dietary Carbohydrate Quantity and Quality in Relation to Risk of Ovulatory Infertility," *European Journal of Clinical Nutrition* 63 (January 2009): 78–86.

11. Robert F. Casper, "Patient Education: Premenstrual Syndrome (PMS) and Premenstrual Dysphoric Disorder (PMDD) (Beyond the Basics)," UpToDate, March 6, 2017, https://www.uptodate.com/contents/premenstrual-syndrome-pms-and-premenstrual-dysphoric-disorder-pmdd-beyond-the-basics.

12. G. E. Abraham, "Nutritional Factors in the Etiology of the Premenstrual Tension Syndromes," *Journal of Reproductive Medicine* 28 (July 1983): 446–464.

13. Audra L. Gollenberg, Mary L. Hediger, Sunni L. Mumford, et al., "Perceived Stress and Severity of Perimenstrual Symptoms: The BioCycle Study," *Journal of Women's Health* 19 (May 2010): 959–967.

14. Jan L. Shifren and Margery L. S. Gass, "The North American Menopause Society Recommendations for Clinical Care of Midlife Women," *Menopause* 21 (October 2014): 1038–1062.

15. S. Pruthi, S. L. Thompson, P. J. Novotny, et al., "Pilot Evaluation of Flaxseed for the Management of Hot Flashes," *Journal of the Society for Integrative Oncology* 5 (Summer 2007): 106–112.

16. D. P. Rose, A. P. Boyar, C. Cohen, and L. E. Strong, "Effect of a Low-Fat Diet on Hormone Levels in Women with Cystic Breast Disease. I. Serum Steroids and Gonadotropins," *Journal of the National Cancer Institute* 78 (April 1987): 623–626.

17. J. F. Dorgan, J. T. Judd, C. Longcope, et al., "Effects of Dietary Fat and Fiber on Plasma and Urine Androgens and Estrogens in Men: A Controlled Feeding Study," *American Journal of Clinical Nutrition* 64 (1996): 850–855.

18. Christina Wang, D. H. Catlin, B. Starcevic, et al., "Low-Fat High-Fiber Diet Decreased Serum and Urine Androgens in Men," *Journal of Clinical Endocrinology & Metabolism* 90 (March 2005): 3550–3559.

19. R. Tamler, "Diabetes, Obesity and Erectile Dysfunction," *Gender Medicine* 6 (2009): 4–16.

20. Cara B. Ebbeling, Janis F. Swain, Henry A. Feldman, et al., "Effects of Dietary Composition during Weight Loss Maintenance: A Controlled Feeding Study," *Journal of the American Medical Association* 307 (June 2012): 2627–2634.

CHAPTER 10 *Keto the Cancer Killer*

1. Centers for Disease Control and Prevention, "Leading Causes of Death," last reviewed March 17, 2017, https://www.cdc.gov/nchs/fastats/leading-causes-of-death.htm.

2. Ophelie Meynet and Jean-Ehrland Ricci, "Caloric Restriction and Cancer: Molecular Mechanisms and Clinical Implications," *Trends in Molecular Medicine* 20 (June 2014): 419–427.

3. S. Koroljow, "Two Cases of Malignant Tumors with Metastases Apparently Treated Successfully with Hypoglycemia Coma," *Psychiatric Quarterly* 36 (1962): 261–270.

4. B. B. Barone, H. C. Yeh, C. F. Snyder, et al., "Long-Term All-Cause Mortality in Cancer Patients with Preexisting Diabetes Mellitus: A Systematic Review and Meta-Analysis," *Journal of the American Medical Association* 300 (December 2008): 2754–2764.

5. Danielle J. Crawley, L. Holmberg, J. C. Melvin, et al., "Serum Glucose and Risk of Cancer: A Meta-Analysis," *BMC Cancer* 14 (December 2014).

6. V. W. Ho, K. Leung, A. Hsu, et al., "A Low Carbohydrate, High Protein Diet Slows Tumor Growth and Prevents Cancer Initiation," *Cancer Research* 71 (July 2011): 4484–4493.

7. Patrick T. Bradshaw, Sharon K. Sagiv, Geoffrey C. Kabat, et al., "Consumption of Sweet Foods and Breast Cancer Risk: A Case-Control Study of Women on Long Island, New York," *Cancer Causes and Control* 20 (October 2009): 1509–1515.

8. C. S. Duchaine, I. Dumas, and C. Diorio, "Consumption of Sweet Foods and Mammographic Breast Density: A Cross-Sectional Study," *BMC Public Health* 14 (June 2014).

9. E. Ax, H. Garmo, B. Grundmark, et al., "Dietary Patterns and Prostate Cancer Risk: Report from the Population Based ULSAM Cohort Study of Swedish Men," *Nutrition and Cancer* 66 (2014): 77–87.

10. A. M. Poff, C. Ari, P. Arnold, T. N. Seyfried, and D. P. D'Agostino, "Ketone Supplementation Decreases Tumor Cell Viability and Prolongs Survival in Mice with Metastatic Cancer," *International Journal of Cancer* 135 (2014): 1711–1720.

11. Sebastian F. Winter, F. Loebel, and J. Dietrich, "Role of Ketogenic Metabolic Therapy in Malignant Glioma: A Systematic Review," *Critical Reviews in Oncology/Hematology* 112 (April 2017): 41–58.

12. Ibid.

13. L. Han, J. Zhang, P. Zhang, et al., "Perspective Research of the Influence of Caloric Restriction Combined with Psychotherapy and Chemotherapy Associated by Hybaroxia on the Prognosis of Patients Suffered by Glioblastoma Multiforme," *Zhonghua Yi Xue Za Zhi* 94 (July 2014): 2129–2131.

14. Winter et al., "Role of Ketogenic Metabolic Therapy in Malignant Glioma."

15. American Cancer Society, "Key Statistics for Colorectal Cancer," last revised February 21, 2018, https://www.cancer.org/cancer/colon-rectal-cancer/about/key-statistics.html.

16. Jeffrey A. Meyerhardt, K. Sato, D. Niedzwiecki, et al., "Dietary Glycemic Load and Cancer Recurrence and Survival in Patients with Stage III Colon Cancer: Findings from CALGB 89803," *Journal of the National Cancer Institute* 104 (November 2012): 1702–1711.

17. Kentaro Nakamura, H. Tonouchi, A. Sasayama, and K. Ashida, "A Ketogenic Formula Prevents Tumor Progression and Cancer Cachexia by Attenuating Systemic Inflammation in Colon 26 Tumor-Bearing Mice," *Nutrients* 10 (February 2018).

18. Eugene J. Fine, C. J. Segal-Isaacson, R. D. Feinman, et al., "Targeting Insulin Inhibition as a Metabolic Therapy in Advanced Cancer: A Pilot Safety and Feasibility Dietary Trial in 10 Patients," *Nutrition* 10 (October 2012): 1028–1035.

19. American Cancer Society, "How Common Is Breast Cancer?" last revised January 4, 2018, https://www.cancer.org/cancer/breast-cancer/about/how-common-is-breast-cancer.html.

20. Ibid.

21. J. J. Branca, S. Pacini, and M. Ruggiero, "Effects of Pre-Surgical Vitamin D Supplementation and Ketogenic Diet in a Patient with Recurrent Breast Cancer," *Anticancer Research* 35 (October 2015): 5525–5532.

22. M. S. Iyikesici, A. K. Slocum, A. Slocum, F. B. Berkarda, M. Kalamian, and T. N. Seyfried, "Efficacy of Metabolically Supported Chemotherapy Combined with Ketogenic

Diet, Hyperthermia and Hyperbaric Oxygen Therapy for Stage IV Triple-Negative Breast Cancer," *Cureus* 9 (July 2017).

23. Yan Jiang, Y. Pan, P. R. Rhea, et al., "A Sucrose-Enriched Diet Promotes Tumorigenesis in Mammary Gland in Part through the 12-Lipoxygenase Pathway," *Cancer Research* 76 (January 2016): 24–29.

24. C. Diorio and I. Dumas, "Relations of Omega-3 and Omega-6 Intake with Mammographic Breast Density," *Cancer Causes and Control* 25 (March 2014): 339–351.

25. American Cancer Society, "Five Ways to Reduce Your Breast Cancer Risk," October 2, 2017, https://www.cancer.org/latest-news/five-ways-to-reduce-your-breast-cancer-risk .html.

26. American Cancer Society, "Key Statistics for Prostate Cancer," last revised January 4, 2018, https://www.cancer.org/cancer/prostate-cancer/about/key-statistics.html.

27. S. J. Freedland, J. Mavropoulos, A. Wang, et al., "Carbohydrate Restriction, Prostate Cancer Growth, and the Insulin-Like Growth Factor Axis," *Prostate* 68 (January 2008): 11–19.

28. Elizabeth M. Masko, J. A. Thomas II, J. A. Antonelli, et al., "Low-Carbohydrate Diets and Prostate Cancer: How Low Is 'Low Enough'?" *Cancer Prevention Research* 3 (September 2010): 1124–1131.

29. Ibid.

30. Melanie Schmidt, N. Pfetzer, M. Schwab, I. Strauss, and U. Kämmerer, "Effects of a Ketogenic Diet on the Quality of Life in 16 Patients with Advanced Cancer: A Pilot Trial," *Nutrition & Metabolism* 8 (July 2011).

31. Mehdi Shakibaei, A. Mobasheri, C. Lueders, F. Busch, P. Shayan, and A. Goel, "Curcumin Enhances the Effect of Chemotherapy against Colorectal Cancer Cells by Inhibition of NF-kB and Src Protein Kinase Signaling Pathways," *PLOS One* 8 (2013).

32. J. M. Lappe, D. Travers-Gustafson, K. M. Davies, R. R. Recker, and R. P. Heaney, "Vitamin D and Calcium Supplementation Reduces Cancer Risk: Results of a Randomized Trial," *American Journal of Clinical Nutrition* 85 (2007): 1586–1591.

CHAPTER 12 *The Keto Fasting Plan*

1. Stephen D. Anton, K. Moehl, W. T. Donahoo, et al., "Flipping the Metabolic Switch: Understanding and Applying Health Benefits of Fasting," *Obesity* 26 (February 2018): 254–268.

2. Shubhroz Gill and Satchidananda Panda, "A Smartphone App Reveals Erratic Diurnal Eating Patterns in Humans That Can Be Modulated for Health Benefits," *Cell Metabolism* 22 (November 2015): 789–798.

3. Valter D. Longo and Satchidananda Panda, "Fasting, Circadian Rhythms, and Time-Restricted Feeding in Healthy Lifespan," *Cell Metabolism* 23 (June 2016): 1048–1059.

CHAPTER 14 *The Keto Collagen-Boosting Plan*

1. E. Proksch, D. Segger, J. Degwert, M. Schunck, V. Zague, and S. Oesser, "Oral Supplementation of Specific Collagen Peptides Has Beneficial Effects on Human Skin Physiology: A Double-Blind, Placebo-Controlled Study," *Skin Pharmacology and Physiology* 27 (2014): 47–55.

2. Maryam Borumand and Sara Sibilla, "Daily Consumption of the Collagen Supplement

Pure Gold Collagen Reduces Visible Signs of Aging," *Clinical Interventions in Aging* 9 (2014): 1747–1758.

3. Misato Yazaki, Y. Ito, M. Yamada, et al., "Oral Ingestion of Collagen Hydrolysate Leads to the Transportation of Highly Concentrated Gly-Pro-Hyp and Its Hydrolyzed Form Pro-Hyp into the Bloodstream and Skin," *Journal of Agricultural and Food Chemistry* 65 (2017): 2315–2322.

4. D. Hexsel, V. Zague, M. Schunck, C. Siega, F. O. Camozzato, and S. Oesser, "Oral Supplementation with Specific Bioactive Collagen Peptides Improves Nail Growth and Symptoms of Brittle Nails," *Journal of Cosmetic Dermatology* 16 (December 2017): 520–526.

5. P. Chen, M. Cescon, and P. Bonaldo, "Lack of Collagen VI Promotes Wound-Induced Hair Growth," *Journal of Investigative Dermatology* 135 (October 2015): 2358–2367.

6. O. Bruyere, B. Zegels, L. Leonori, et al., "Effect of Collagen Hydrolysate in Articular Pain: A 6-Month Randomized, Double-Blind Placebo Controlled Study," *Complementary Therapies in Medicine* 20 (June 2012): 124–130.

7. K. L. Clark, W. Sebastianelli, K. R. Flechsenhar, et al., "24-Week Study on the Use of Collagen Hydrolysate as a Dietary Supplement in Athletes with Activity-Related Joint Pain," *Current Medical Research and Opinion* 24 (May 2008): 1485–1496.

8. D. E. Trentham, R. A. Dynesius-Trentham, E. J. Orav, et al., "Effects of Oral Administration of Type II Collagen on Rheumatoid Arthritis," *Science* 261 (September 1993): 1727–1730.

CHAPTER 15 *The Keto Cancer Plan*

1. American Cancer Society, "Study: Cancer Patients with Strong Religious or Spiritual Beliefs Report Better Health," October 21, 2015, https://www.cancer.org/latest -news/study-cancer-patients-with-strong-religious-or-spiritual-beliefs-report -better-health.html.

2. Heather S. L. Jim, J. E. Pustejovsky, C. L. Park, et al., "Religion, Spirituality, and Physical Health in Cancer Patients: A Meta-Analysis," *Cancer* 121 (November 2015): 3760–3768.

3. Jacqui Stringer, R. Swindell, and M. Dennis, "Massage in Patients Undergoing Intensive Chemotherapy Reduces Serum Cortisol and Prolactin," *Psycho-Oncology* 10 (October 2008): 1024–1031.

4. M.P. Bennett, J. M. Zeller, L. Rosenberg, and J. McCann, "The Effect of Mirthful Laughter on Stress and Natural Killer Cell Activity," *Alternative Therapies in Health and Medicine* 9 (March–April 2003): 38–45.

Index

About the Author

Dr. Josh Axe, DNM, DC, CNS, is the founder of the world's #1 most visited natural health website, DrAxe.com. He is also the bestselling author of *Eat Dirt* and the cofounder of the Ancient Nutrition supplement company. Dr. Axe appears regularly on *The Dr. Oz Show* and has written for *Shape, PopSugar, HuffPost, Men's Health, Forbes, Business Insider, Muscle & Fitness Hers,* and *Well+Good*.